W9-BRX-287

THE AMERICAN YOGA ASSOCIATION'S

Easy Does It® Yoga

The Safe and Gentle Way to Health and Well-Being

ALICE CHRISTENSEN

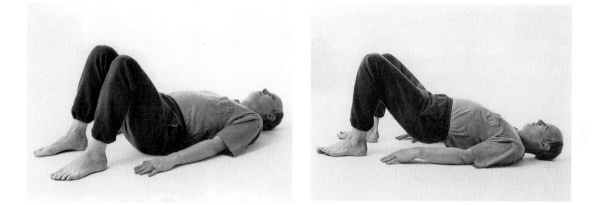

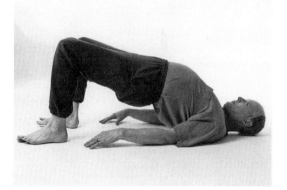

AMERICAN
Y·O·G·A
ASSOCIATION

A Fireside Book
Published by Simon & Schuster

FIRESIDE
Rockefeller Center
1230 Avenue of the Americas
New York, NY 10020

Easy Does It® Yoga is a trademark of the
American Yoga Association

FIRESIDE and colophon are registered trademarks
of Simon & Schuster, Inc.

Photographs by Evelyn England and Herbert Ascherman, Jr.
Designed by Diane Hobbing

Manufactured in the United States of America
10 9 8 7 6 5 4 3 2 1

Library of Congress Cataloging-in-Publication Data
Christensen, Alice.
     The American Yoga Association's easy does it yoga :
the safe and gentle way to health and well-being /
Alice Christensen.
        p.   cm.
     Includes Index.
     1. Yoga, Hatha.   2. Yoga—Health aspects.
I. American Yoga Association.   II. Title.   III. Title:
Easy does it yoga.
RA781.7.C52   1999
613.7'046—dc21   99-39751
                                                    CIP

ISBN 0-684-84890-2

ACKNOWLEDGMENTS

My deepest appreciation goes to the staff, students, and friends of the American Yoga Association, who contributed to this book in so many invaluable ways.

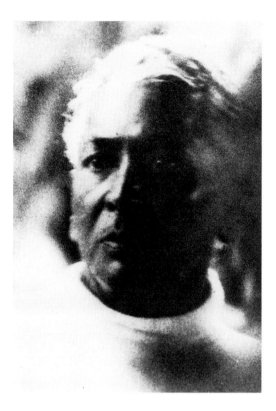

Swami Rama (1900–1972)
of Kashmir and Haridwar, India

This book is dedicated to a remarkable man: my teacher, Rama. One of the world's greatest masters of Yoga, he embodied the noblest aspirations of humanity: He was a scholar, writer, poet, musician, psychologist, philosopher, diplomat, and loving, supportive teacher. He was unassuming and humble, yet his greatness shone through all the facets of his personality and illuminated the lives of everyone who knew him.

It is my memory of him, what he taught me, and the excellence of what he represented that are the energy and source of this book. He was the ideal example of a happy and wise older individual who is capable of inspiring and guiding younger generations. Rama was sixty-two years old when he first came to this country and we met for the first time. I can still remember his golden complexion, unforgettable eyes, and tremendous strength and vitality. Despite his age, he could outthink and even outrun me. He was a powerful testimony to the value of Yoga for anyone.

Through Yoga, Rama was able to take the harshest of life's sorrows and the finest of its joys and make use of each for growth and wisdom. He inspired me to strive for this same ability to rise above any despair and to make full use of every experience in life. I never forget what he told me: "Yoga makes the rough road smooth."

I learned from Rama that my life, my body, and my mind were created to grow and mature in wisdom throughout my entire life. Through my practice of Yoga, I was able to use these new ideas and become more aware of my inner self. I studied all the philosophy I could get my hands on, especially the many different perspectives on life and death. I was particularly touched by the Bhagavad Gita, which describes the inner self like this: "As a man discarding worn-out clothes takes others which are new, likewise the embodied soul, casting off worn-out bodies, enters into others which are new. Weapons cannot cut it, nor can fire burn it; water cannot drench it, nor can wind make it dry."

It was not until I had an experience during meditation of slipping out of my body that I really saw the truth of what Rama had said to me. I suddenly found myself looking down at my body. It was still there, on the floor, but I was looking at it from high above. I knew then that no matter how dear to me my limited concept of myself was, it was not the total picture at all.

Rama taught me that our later years are the sum and

substance of how we live when we are young. Ethical behavior then has meaning, because these disciplines give us solace and strength as we get older.

It is the light of this great man's genius, the light of Yoga, that shines from the pages of this book. He was a truly exceptional man who had more capacity for love, knowledge, joy, insight, and beauty than I could ever imagine.

CONTENTS

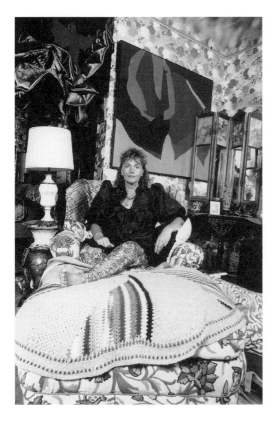

PREFACE

The Easy Does It Yoga (EDY) program began in Cleveland, Ohio, in 1964. I had studied Yoga for many years by then and had just returned from an extended period of seclusion in India with my teacher, Rama. When I arrived to teach my very first Yoga class, I was surprised to find that all the students were over sixty years old. One said, "We didn't tell you how old we were on the phone because we thought if you knew we were all grandparents, you wouldn't come." They, as well as most other Americans in those days, had the mistaken idea that Yoga was an exotic kind of exercise meant only for young bodies. I saw for the first time in this class of brave beginners that many of the problems that robbed them of their health, vitality, and independence could be reversed. Many of their chronic health problems and negative attitudes toward themselves and growing old simply disappeared.

One class of seniors followed another, and the benefits to their health, appearance, and self-esteem became obvious. A remarkable transformation was taking place. Where there had been stiff and painful joints, there was now the spring of a more youthful step. Instead of a grim, depressed, defeated attitude, there was now joy and interest in life once again. Most important, my students were able to regain their self-respect and the respect of others with their mental clarity and emotional stability. My students were throwing off the rejection and fear engendered by their advancing years and were beginning to take their rightful place in society.

These observations were intensified when I visited my parents, who were living in a large trailer park in Florida. Living in close proximity to so many older people exposed me to many of the problems experienced by both Sunbelt retirees and the rural elderly of Florida's farm communities. I realized that these older people in Florida had the same problems as my older students in Cleveland, and that the program that I had developed in Cleveland could be tremendously effective in helping older people everywhere live happier, healthier, and more productive lives.

With a small group of students, I founded the American Yoga Association (then called the Light of Yoga

Society) in 1969. Easy Does It Yoga was an important part of our curriculum from the beginning, and it soon began to earn local and national recognition for its many benefits. We published the first edition of *Easy Does It Yoga* in 1975 as demand for information about Yoga for seniors increased. Our teaching staff began giving free introductory classes in Easy Does It Yoga to any interested group. In just three years, over ten thousand people attended these free classes at more than two hundred locations in Ohio, Florida, and neighboring states.

The culmination of our work occurred when we were invited to apply for a federal grant for teaching Easy Does It Yoga throughout the Tampa Bay area on Florida's Gulf Coast. A scientifically controlled study of this program's effectiveness was a part of that exciting program. In the decade that followed, we were able to bring the techniques of Easy Does It Yoga to many urban and rural populations of seniors through several federal, state, local, and private grants, many of which included additional research studies.

From the results of these studies and our own continuing observations, we realized that Easy Does It Yoga can also be of tremendous help to people of any age who are physically challenged due to chronic illness, recovery from substance abuse, hardening of the arteries and other manifestations of heart disease, obesity, convalescence from illness, or recovery from injury. In the past twenty years, Easy Does It Yoga has been used by physical therapists, nurses, home health aides, and family members to help their clients and loved ones regain and maintain independence, enabling them to live longer, healthier, and stronger lives.

Easy Does It Yoga has come a long way since those first classes in 1964. As someone who is nearing the age of seventy, I now realize more than ever how important it is to remain fit and independent; I rely on Yoga to help me maintain a happy, vigorous outlook on life as I get older and to keep me healthy and strong while I enjoy my older years. I wish you the same success as you begin your practice of Easy Does It Yoga.

Alice Christensen
October 1998
Sarasota, Florida

INTRODUCTION:

Yoga and Your Lifestyle

"Doing this Yoga every day has made me a changed person. I feel so alive now that I just want to do things. I used to feel sluggish and fatigued. I'd just as soon lie on the davenport and just sleep or nap, rather than doing anything. Now, oh heavens, you wouldn't believe what a changed person I am! Now I go disco dancing every Wednesday and Thursday. Not in my wildest dreams would I have thought that I would ever have the energy to go out and do these things. It's just grand!"

—Jeanne Hrovat (age 66)

Most of us know that in order to maintain health, we need regular exercise. However, if you are elderly, convalescing from an illness, recovering from an injury or from substance abuse, or if you simply haven't exercised in many years, you may be hesitant—not knowing where to begin, or even afraid to exercise for fear of hurting yourself. Easy Does It Yoga is a safe, gentle program that any adult can do. Its greatest value is that you will love it. It will not become a burden; rather, it will help lift your spirits and become a happy support for everyday living. Easy Does It Yoga is a complete fitness program in itself. It can help you build strength as well as the confidence to engage in more vigorous exercise, if you wish.

Easy Does It Yoga is a holistic program of simple exercise, breathing, relaxation, and meditation techniques designed to help you regain and maintain health, well-being, and independence. The program also includes some discussions about philosophy, to stretch your mental muscles, and up-to-date nutritional guidelines to help you make informed choices about what you eat. The practice of Easy Does It Yoga encourages a positive view of aging and physical capabilities because it shows you that you need not be limited by these conditions. Easy Does It Yoga can help you live your life to the fullest. It is a program that fits the expression "If I knew then what I know now . . . ," giving you the choice to have a wholesome, healthy body that makes for a wonderful, productive life.

Easy Does It Yoga is derived from the classical techniques of Yoga, which date back more than five thousand years. In ancient times, the desire for greater personal freedom, longer life, and heightened self-understanding gave birth to this system of physical and mental exercise that has since spread throughout the world.

The whole school of Yoga is built on three main structures: exercise, breathing, and meditation. Yoga exercises are designed to put pressure on the glandular systems of the body, thereby increasing its efficiency and total health. The body is looked upon as the primary instrument that enables us to work and evolve in the world, and so a Yoga student treats it with great care and respect. Breathing techniques are based on the concept that breath is the source of life in the body. The Yoga student gently increases breath control to improve the health and function of both body and mind. These two systems of exercise and breathing then prepare the body and mind for meditation, and the student finds an easy approach to a quiet mind that allows silence and healing of the damage caused by everyday stress. Regular daily practice of all three parts of Yoga produces a clear, bright mind and a strong, capable body.

"Yoga" is a Sanskrit word that means "to join" or "to yoke," and the practice of Yoga brings the body and mind together into one harmonious experience. It might surprise you to learn that traditionally, the ideal age to begin the practice of Yoga was said to be fifty-three, the age marking one's passage into a new stage of life, one of contemplation and self-discovery. Yoga was traditionally practiced by older people and was designed to develop better physical and mental health.

Easy Does It Yoga will show you that exercise does not have to be strenuous, painful, or boring. Once you find out how enjoyable it is to practice Easy Does It Yoga, you will be able to overcome one of the most problematic factors in the American lifestyle: inactivity.

Inactivity is a habit—a habit that is easy to fall into as we get older and extra movement becomes stressful. If you have been sick, it can be difficult and uncomfortable even to think about moving around actively again. The desire to become strong and well is sometimes blocked by the hopeless attitude "I can never do it. It takes too much effort. I'm not worth anything." When you practice Easy Does It Yoga, you can cure that problem by immediately improving your self-confidence and enjoyment of life.

In this day and age, there are always more ways to make life easier for ourselves. Almost anything can be purchased by mail order, for example; even food can be delivered right to our doorstep. The problem with such conveniences is that they help to create a lifestyle that is more and more sedentary. A typical weekday for many of us may involve rising from a comfortable mattress after a full night's sleep, driving to work, sitting at a desk most of the day, driving home, and relaxing all evening on a couch or in an easy chair until it's time for bed again. Our most common entertainments are other sedentary pastimes such as videotapes, movies, concerts, and spectator sports. If you are among those fortunate enough to take advantage of the luxuries of mail order, the latest labor-saving devices, and other comforts, you still need an inner courage and impetus to stay well and strong by continuing to exercise. Otherwise, a sedentary lifestyle can make you vulnerable to many chronic health problems.

The sedentary lifestyle eats away quietly and steadily at physical and mental health. Without exercise, muscle turns to fat, circulation slows down, fat clogs artery walls, and the brain gets less oxygen. It becomes harder to get out of bed or the easy chair. We tire more easily and sometimes even become depressed. Energy levels fall, and so we reduce our activity even more.

Inactivity can be directly associated with many of the problems that are usually attributed to aging or illness, such as stiffness, overweight, constipation, back pain, high blood pressure, depression, anxiety, and insomnia. Inactive people spend more weeks bedridden, visit doctors more often, have a lower opinion of their health, and die younger than do those who maintain an active lifestyle. Most people who gain weight in midlife and their older years do so not because of overeating but because of decreased activity levels.

Our sedentary lifestyle catches up with us when, for some reason, we fall out of even minimal exercise habits, when we're injured, for example, or recovering from a major illness. Perhaps office politics, financial needs, or other motivations lead us to value our work more than our health. Major life changes, such as retirement, children leaving home, or moving to a new home, can also disrupt our regular activity levels, as can the onset of chronic illness.

> "I started taking Yoga so I could be involved in some type of exercising activity. You see, for seventeen years I indulged in high-impact aerobics. However, in 1996 I had an attack that was diagnosed as multiple sclerosis (MS). I was only forty-four at the time, and I knew I needed to do something. Yoga has helped me focus on the breathing and stretching aspect, allowing me to relieve some stressful situations occurring in everyday life. Even though I can't do every exercise, the ones I can do give me a sense of accomplishment."
> —Barbara Solomon (age 47)

Inactivity can cause people of any age to experience difficulty coping with stress. Sometimes people begin to use alcohol or drugs to escape the feelings of depression and anxiety that are common results of inactivity. Easy Does It Yoga exercise provides a constant, safe release for feelings of stress. A few minutes of daily practice prevent everyday stresses from accumulating to levels that can bring on depression and anxiety.

Anyone who has ever experienced a serious injury, illness, or addiction knows that it takes a long time to recover. Even after a simple cold, sometimes it takes weeks before we feel like ourselves again. Often a longer time passes before we feel like exercising.

The habit of inactivity is pervasive even without the disabling effects of an illness or injury. Many of us do some form of exercise for fun: We might play a set of tennis on the weekend, or swim a few laps on a hot day. Few people, however, exercise with the regularity and the vigor necessary to get really fit and stay that way. We all know it would be better to exercise more, but we find that we really don't want to. It seems like such an effort! It is easy to find all sorts of excuses for not exercising when your exercise program is dull and boring: "In the morning, I'm too stiff." "During the day, I'm too busy." "In the evening, I'm too tired from working all day." "It hurts too much." "I have a bad knee." "I don't have the right shoes." "It's raining."

The quality and amount of exercise you get every day can be the single most important factor in maintaining your good health, and with Easy Does It Yoga, you can exercise properly in as little as five minutes. The hardest part of any new fitness program is getting started. Easy Does It Yoga is such an enjoyable program that it won't have you looking for excuses. It will give you the motivation to take up a daily exercise program with vigor and delight.

Health professionals agree that for many chronic health problems, the best treatment is to change the lifestyle patterns that contribute to the symptoms. For example, several recent studies have proven that a combination of Yoga exercise and meditation and a low-fat diet can actually reverse heart disease. Adult-onset diabetes is another example of a chronic illness that can often be reversed when you pay careful attention to diet and practice moderate exercise such as that provided by the Easy Does It Yoga program.

In Easy Does It Yoga you will find a way to coax your body and mind toward health and vitality by using gentle, safe, interesting, and enjoyable movements that can be done easily—even if you are currently bedridden. You don't need any special equipment or clothing, and you can practice almost anywhere, anytime: watching television, standing in line at the store, or even lying in bed. The program includes exercise, breathing, and relaxation techniques that you will love. These techniques will gradually increase your stamina, strength, flexibility, and feelings of well-being. I can assure you that you will notice a definite improvement within one week if you practice a few minutes each day.

Many people associate Yoga primarily with stretching and relaxation, and most people who take Yoga classes do so for stress management, to learn how to relax, or to increase flexibility. These benefits definitely exist. However, there is a more subtle, cumulative effect of regular Yoga practice that directly affects mood and self-awareness, and it is this aspect that confronts—and defeats—the moodiness, isolation, and depression caused by inactivity. Because of its efficient, specialized movements, controlled breathing, and relaxation training, Yoga acts very quickly to help you maintain a centered, positive attitude. If a Yoga class is taught correctly, no one leaves tired, depressed, or worn out. It is not a competitive program. Instead, you will learn to adjust it specifically to your own needs.

> *"A friend of mine teaches Yoga and asked me to help her review the Easy Does It Yoga curriculum. She knew I wasn't an active person and didn't like to exercise because I have a bad shoulder and back problem. She assured me that Easy Does It Yoga wasn't too strenuous and that the exercises could be modified if I found them too difficult. I found that I could do most everything and I wasn't in pain. After we did exercises every day for several days, I found I was beginning to enjoy my new pain-free shoulder and back, thanks to Easy Does It Yoga."*
> —Terry Lewis (age 65)

As you begin, it will be easy to master the simple movements and techniques of Easy Does It Yoga. Even a little daily practice will show increasing benefits each day. I suggest that you begin by trying just five minutes of Easy Does It Yoga twice a day. You can choose the exercises and breathing techniques that you like best. You won't find it tiresome or boring, and you will notice an immediate sense of well-being that will encourage you to practice a little longer each day. I believe that twenty minutes is sufficient for a complete, entirely beneficial exercise session. If you want to add a relaxation/meditation session, begin with ten minutes and then gradually add more time if you wish.

Whatever your physical condition, you can use Easy Does It Yoga to improve the quality of your life. It will empower you to do the things that you want to do to make your life happy, healthy, and rewarding.

CHAPTER 1

The Easy Does It Yoga Program of Total Fitness: How It Works and What to Expect

"Since my physical limitations have curtailed most of my activities, I really have a psychological need to feel like I'm accomplishing something or I get despondent and depressed. Improving my physical abilities in my Yoga helps give me that needed sense of accomplishment."

—Dorothy Wild (age 69)

Each aspect of Easy Does It Yoga training engages different parts of your body and mind. There are five major parts to the Easy Does It Yoga program:

- *Exercises:* Gentle stretching, strengthening, and balancing movements that can be done in a chair, in bed, in a pool, in a wheelchair, or on the floor.
- *Breathing Techniques:* Slow, diaphragmatic breathing techniques that strengthen the respiratory and circulatory systems.
- *Relaxation and Meditation:* Step-by-step procedures that release tension throughout the body, improve concentration, increase circulation to the heart, and brighten mood.
- *Nutrition:* Suggestions for building health by gradually improving diet.
- *Philosophy:* Ideas from Yoga philosophy that enhance creative thought, promote inner growth, and stimulate intuition.

"Since I started Yoga I feel so much more energetic, alive, and alert. And you know, it's the combination of everything in this Yoga, not just one thing, that did it—it's the whole thing."

—Jeanne Hrovat (age 66)

EXERCISE

Easy Does It Yoga modifies traditional Yoga exercises into a safe, gentle, and gradual system that does not require great limberness or stamina and is noncompetitive. Easy Does It Yoga exercises consist of nonstrenuous bends, lifts, and twists performed with specific breathing patterns. They can be done while you are standing, seated in a chair or wheelchair, in bed, or in a bathtub or pool. I encourage you to do them at any odd time of day, while you watch television in your favorite chair, stand in line, or wait in your car, for example. These exercises, or some variation of them, can be done by anyone, regardless of physical limitations.

If you have been inactive or ill for a long time, do not allow yourself to think that you are too stiff or disabled to begin exercising again. Even if you are very weak, blind, recovering from an injury, severely disabled, or suffering with addiction, you can now benefit from regular exercise that you will love and that will be easy for you to do. Many studies, as well as our own experiences with students over the past forty years, have undeniably proven that the participants who have been the least active and who are the most damaged by inactivity have benefited the most from this exercise program.

Any exercise program needs to be enjoyable—otherwise you will not continue doing it. Many of us say we hate to exercise, but you will love doing Easy Does It Yoga exercises. After doing your exercise program each day, you will not be tired, but instead will feel refreshed, energized, and bright. Our students give the best testimony to the fact that they enjoy Easy Does It Yoga: On the average, they practice their exercises ten minutes longer every day than we suggest!

The physical and mental benefits of Easy Does It Yoga exercise include:

- *Increased mobility:* Loosens stiff, frozen joints; strengthens and limbers the muscles, tendons, and ligaments.
- *Improved circulation:* Increases blood supply to head, arms, and legs; normalizes blood pressure; eases the strain on the heart.
- *Increased respiratory strength:* Strengthens breathing muscles; loosens the chest wall; restores elasticity of lung tissue.
- *Improved health in digestive and genitourinary systems:* Stimulates smooth muscle tone of digestive and eliminative organs by deep internal massage to deal with constipation, bladder, and prostate problems; improves sexual function; relieves incontinence.
- *More energy and zest for life:* Restores self-confidence; improves self-esteem; increases energy for daily tasks.
- *Better weight control:* Relieves depression and anxiety that trigger overeating; strengthens the will to eat correctly and exercise regularly.
- *Better coordination:* Restores body awareness; improves balance; strengthens the nerves that control body movement.
- *Reduced anxiety and loneliness:* Reduces fear and nervousness by releasing tensions and frustrations that build up in the body and mind; builds a better self-image; builds the strength to enjoy a more outgoing lifestyle; rebuilds self-confidence.

"The deep breathing has helped me to relax tremendously. I sleep better if I do my deep breathing every day. Sometimes I used to go for four or five nights with very little sleep—that's murder. I was getting really depressed from a lack of sleep. But now my Yoga relaxes me so much that I not only sleep better at night, but I can nap in the afternoon, which I hadn't been able to do in years."

—Helen Gould (age 64)

BREATHING TECHNIQUES

Breathing techniques are one of the most helpful aspects of Easy Does It Yoga. Attention to breathing can add years to your life as well as greatly improving the quality of your life right now. Breath is vital for life, yet, perhaps because breathing is so automatic, we often give it little consideration. Unless we are faced with a serious respiratory condition such as asthma, emphysema, bronchitis, or pneumonia, we take our breathing for granted.

Most people breathe with only the upper third of their lungs, resulting in an inefficient exchange of oxygen and other gases in the body. The breathing exercises in Easy Does It Yoga retrain your body to use your lungs to their fullest capacity. Many of our students tell us that breathing exercises are their favorite part of the course, and they do them while watching television, walking, bathing, or even lying in bed. Breathing techniques can be used to lessen insomnia and to reduce the effects of upsetting emotions such as anxiety or anger. They can also help regulate blood pressure. Some of the common problems associated with aging, such as confusion, memory loss, depression, and fatigue, can also be helped by your learning to breathe more deeply.

Here's why: Inactivity contributes to the pattern of breathing more with the upper lung area than the lower, and this condition tends to worsen with age. Unfortunately, the blood vessels that pick up the oxygen accumulate more in the lower lung. As a result, the oxygen content of the blood tends to decrease with age. Since the brain requires three times as much oxygen as the rest of the body, it is affected most severely by lower blood levels of oxygen. This decreased oxygen level contributes to the confused, muddled thinking that sometimes accompanies aging. Lung efficiency normally decreases further when you lie down; nighttime confusion—a common condition in which people wake during the night momentarily unable to remember where or who they are—frequently results from a decrease in oxygen levels during sleep. The sluggish, depressed moods of many of our students disappear when they begin to breathe better. If you feel depressed upon waking, it may simply be due to reduced oxygen flow to your brain during the night.

Strengthening the muscles in the diaphragm and the abdomen brings each breath lower into the lungs where more of the blood circulates. You will learn to breathe easier, deeper, and slower, getting more of the fresh energy of life to the brain and body. You will enjoy life more because your mind is brighter and more alert.

Some of the physical and mental benefits of Easy Does It Yoga breathing techniques are:

- *Increased strength:* Increases the strength of all the muscles and nerves used in breathing, including the diaphragm and the muscles between the ribs; strengthens back muscles; increases vigor.
- *Greater limberness:* Increases the flexibility of the joints where the ribs join the breastbone in the front and the spine in the back.
- *Greater vital capacity:* Increases the volume of air that one can breathe.
- *Increased oxygen and energy levels:* Increases the amount of oxygen available to all parts of the body, raising energy levels.
- *Easier breathing:* Lowers the respiration rate by deepening the air flow into the total lung space.
- *Reduced heart strain:* Decreasing the number of breaths per minute and increasing oxygen supply reduces strain on the heart, helping to normalize blood pressure.

"You can make yourself sick just by thinking, and a lot of these older people today, they get so despondent they just quit living. But not me—I got it—I get the benefit of this Yoga. Just don't overdo, that's all. Build up slowly and keep going, and sure enough you'll be compensated for your efforts. You'll feel more alive."

—Gene Roy (age 62)

RELAXATION AND MEDITATION

Relaxation is a valuable tool that helps you eliminate accumulated tension and strain. Easy Does It Yoga teaches you how to visualize tension spots in different parts of your body and gently relax them. You can do this either sitting in a chair or lying in bed or on the floor. Practice the technique at various times during the day. It's especially useful when you are watching television or waiting for an appointment.

After you completely relax your body, meditation training takes over to relax and quiet your mind. This produces a state of deep silence and peace. Both of these practices improve concentration skills, memory, and self-esteem.

Some of the physical and mental benefits of relaxation and meditation training include:

- *Less tension and stress:* Shows you how to quiet your mind and relax tension in the body without medicine; helps to normalize blood pressure.
- *Improved concentration and awareness:* Increases alertness and willpower; develops intuition.
- *Increased coping skills:* Teaches you how to tolerate stress and create a more balanced outlook on daily frustrations.
- *Reduced anxiety, irritability, and nervousness:* Shows you how to change your moods if you wish.
- *Reduced dependence on medications or alcohol:* Encourages you to systematically relax yourself so you don't need to rely so much on self-medication.
- *A positive self-image:* Improves your view of yourself; stimulates creative thought and intuition.
- *Diminished fears:* Develops greater freedom from incapacitating fears, and shows you how to explore your full potential.
- *Openness to new views:* Develops sensitivity to your inner being; creates greater feelings of connection to others and the world around you; provides strength and encouragement for you to explore your own ideas about life and your relationship to the world.

"This Yoga was a blessing from God for me. I had been through seven operations and was on twenty-six pills a day for pain and depression. You name it. I told the doctor, 'Hey, I can't live like this. I've got to do something.' He said, 'Double the dose.' I came and told my wife, Mary, 'That's it.' I dumped all the pills in the toilet and flushed it. That was five years ago. I was so determined to be out of that condition. When I started this Yoga exercise there was some pain, sure, but nothing like what I'd already been through. Before this Yoga I never did any exercise at all. Now, hey, I feel so good. It's helped give me back ninety-nine and three-fourths percent of my life. I'm a new person!"

—Gene Roy (age 62)

NUTRITION

Many Americans eat a diet that is imbalanced and deficient in many essential nutrients. Our high-sugar, high-fat, and low-fiber diet is prematurely killing us. Overconsumption of saturated fats, cholesterol, sugar, salt, and alcohol has been correlated with six of the ten leading causes of death: heart disease, cancer, cerebrovascular disease, diabetes, arteriosclerosis, and cirrhosis of the liver. Making the problem worse, often older adults are especially attracted to high-fat, high-sugar diets because diminished senses of taste and smell make rich foods more appealing.

People of any age who feel listless and depressed due to inactivity, substance abuse, or convalescence tend to eat what is convenient and comforting rather than what is nutritious. Weight is also an increasing problem: Recent surveys show that over 40 percent of adults in the United States are overweight to a degree that may impair health and longevity. Underweight, and associated loss of appetite, are also a problem in some people. Both of these problems of imbalance can be corrected with proper nutrition.

Conditions such as obesity, osteoporosis, diabetes, arthritis, cardiovascular disease, anemia, constipation, and many nonspecific complaints such as confusion, poor appetite, melancholy, and listlessness can be improved when you change your diet following the guidelines in this book.

The nutritional suggestions that follow present an attractive alternative to our unhealthy American diet. Our suggestions are based on choosing more traditional foods—foods that are less processed and with fewer added chemicals—and preparing them more simply. Far from being a new "health food" diet, these suggestions resemble the way we ate before food technology became such a big business. In this book you will find a flexible diet substantially lower in fats and higher in unrefined carbohydrates than the average American diet. A diet higher in fresh or frozen fruits, vegetables, and grains and lower in processed or refined foods is healthier, cheaper, and lower in calories.

You will achieve a better diet as you learn:

• How to recognize and purchase nutritious foods on a limited income.
• How to store and prepare foods for best nutritional value.
• How to recognize the most common nutritional diseases and what to do about them.
• How to supplement your diet wisely.

PHILOSOPHY

Yoga is not based on any original book or scripture; instead, its precepts have been handed down orally from teacher to student for thousands of years. The goal of this philosophy is self-understanding and the development of a harmoniously balanced individual. The essence of Yoga philosophy is transformation.

The ideas and growth associated with Yoga have tremendous value for everyone. As you begin to know yourself better, your self-esteem and leadership abilities emerge. You will ultimately discover something at the very core of your being that does not change, or grow old. In Yoga this is called the Self, and it is considered to be the real support of the individual. As self-awareness grows, you become more resistant to the negative attitudes of depression, fear, and despair that are often associated with age or disability, and you will be able to find a deep beauty, contentment, and balance inside yourself.

Practicing Easy Does It Yoga philosophy will result in benefits such as:

- Increased self-respect and positive self-image, along with greater tolerance of others.
- Enhanced, more mature concepts of life and death; happiness with genuine appreciation in later stages of life.

"As my strength and control of my body have improved, I have a feeling of physical well-being, which gives impetus to a greater participation in recreational and social activities. My family and friends have commented favorably on the change in my personal appearance. This gives a lift to my mental outlook, which, in turn, results in a feeling of emotional well-being. The Yoga philosophy and meditation also lead to a spiritual well-being and self-acceptance—an acceptance of one's own years and that we are worthwhile, with contributions yet to make in life."
—Harriet Peel (age 74)

CHAPTER 2

Getting Started

"I'm a double amputee, and I get tired of just sitting around doing nothing. I really look forward to my Easy Does It Yoga. I practice at least four to five days a week and it makes me feel good. The breathing, relaxation, and exercises make me feel stronger and useful, and it's very nice. I enjoy it a lot!"

—Buster Henderson (age 47)

Before you begin learning the Easy Does It Yoga techniques, here are some commonsense suggestions to keep you safe and help you use this book most effectively.

YOUR DAILY SCHEDULE

In order to get the best results, you should include in your daily routine a few minutes each of exercise, breathing techniques, and meditation. Start with these suggested times and increase them whenever you wish:

Exercise—10 minutes
Breathing—5 minutes
Meditation—10 minutes

If you are unable at first to practice 25 minutes per day, start with just 5 minutes once or twice during the day. Try to practice a little of each type of technique; for instance, in just 5 minutes you can practice three exercises, breathe in and out three times, and sit quietly for a minute or two in relaxation. Even a little daily practice will bring results.

Of course, you can practice your exercises and other techniques at any time of day as well, such as while listening to the radio, talking on the telephone, or waiting in cars or offices. This is the best way to truly integrate Easy Does It Yoga into your daily life. Many people, for example, practice seated exercises such as leg lifts or knee squeezes in front of the television, or the Complete Breath while waiting for an appointment.

Don't forget the chapters on nutrition and philosophy. Each week, try to improve your diet in one small way, and pick one philosophical concept to think about or a book from the reading list to read and discuss with friends.

You will find a suggested six-week curriculum incorporating all five aspects of Easy Does It Yoga in the next chapter, which also includes suggested routines for bed and wheelchair.

ALWAYS CHECK WITH YOUR DOCTOR

Before beginning any new exercise program, talk to your doctor. Take this book with you and ask your doctor if there are any movements that you should be especially careful with at first. Most physicians are happy to see their patients taking an interest in improving their own health and will gladly work with you to design a routine that will accommodate any limitations you have. You will find some special notes on Yoga for different health conditions later in this chapter.

USE YOUR COMMON SENSE

If you haven't exercised in a long time, or if you are recovering from an illness, start slowly. Sometimes, in their zeal to feel better, people overdo. These exercises are designed to work very efficiently, so you don't need to exceed the recommended number of repetitions (usually three). If you feel stiff or sore the day after exercising, you have pushed yourself too hard. You should not feel any pain or discomfort as a result of practicing Easy Does It Yoga.

EATING AND DRINKING

Wait one to two hours after eating a heavy meal before you start exercising. You will have better success with breathing and meditation if you wait an hour or so after drinking coffee, tea, cola, or other caffeine-containing beverages. Never practice Yoga under the influence of alcohol.

PLACE AND TIME

You will have the best success if you try to practice your routine at the same time every day. Even a small daily commitment to 5, 10, or 15 minutes will start the momentum that will steadily increase your benefits from Yoga. Practice the techniques throughout the day as well, whenever you feel like it. Some people like to do their routine first thing in the morning to give their day a jump start. Others prefer to practice in the early evening to help them relax after a hectic day. Whatever time of day you choose, the important thing is to do something at least once in every 24-hour period. This will give you the best, fastest results.

Practice in a room that is private and reasonably quiet. Turn off your telephone and keep pets in another room. Ask your family to give you a few minutes of uninterrupted time for your Yoga practice, especially during your meditation. The temperature of the room should be comfortable; avoid cold drafts and stay as warm as possible.

CLOTHING AND EQUIPMENT

Wear loose, warm clothing for Yoga practice. Avoid belts and constricting garments. Try to practice the exercises in bare feet, and put on a pair of socks for your meditation. During meditation, your body gets so relaxed that your body temperature will naturally drop, so avoid getting chilled; throw a sweater or shawl around you during your relaxation and meditation period. Wrapping yourself also provides a psychological feeling of protection for the quiet, vulnerable period of meditation.

Choose a mat, blanket, or beach towel to do your floor exercises on, and keep that mat separate; use it only for Yoga. If it is not large enough for your entire body to rest on it, be sure to rest your head on it, especially during meditation if you are meditating lying down.

For exercises done in a chair, use a straight, sturdy chair. For standing balance exercises, stand near a counter or use the back of a sturdy chair for support.

OTHER HELPFUL HINTS

The special binding of this book allows you to lay it flat on the floor or a table so you can refer to it often as you exercise. The symbols beside each exercise show which ones can be done in bed ⬛, wheelchair ♿, or pool 🏊. If you exercise in a pool, do the seated exercises sitting on a step, and standing exercises holding on to a ledge or railing for support.

Read the instructions for each exercise all the way through before you try it. Move slowly and carefully as you are practicing Yoga exercises; never bounce or jerk in any of the movements in Yoga. Be sure to follow the breathing patterns exactly as instructed for each exercise, and always breathe through your nose. A warm bath or shower before practicing will help relax your muscles and loosen your joints. Massage your joints frequently during your exercise routine to help keep them limber and warm (see pp. 72–74).

If you are ill, you can still practice your breathing exercises and meditation while resting in bed, and you can even do some easy exercises such as the Foot Flap and Ankle Rotation (p. 81), Elbow

Touch (p. 66), and Shoulder Roll (p. 67). Be careful not to overdo. Practice the Complete Breath (p. 58) whenever you think of it. Try to keep eating a balanced, healthy diet.

"I used to be really stiff. The arthritis settled in the front of my legs all the way down to my toes. It got so that I couldn't lift my feet. I had to slide them across the floor in order to get around. Now, since I started doing my Yoga leg exercises, I can not only lift my feet, but I can move my whole leg and get around by myself again."

—Emma Mae Mays (age 62)

YOGA FOR CHRONIC HEALTH CONDITIONS

The exercises and other techniques in this book are designed so that almost anyone can do them. If you have one or more chronic health conditions, however, you may need some special advice. Here are the Easy Does It Yoga techniques that might be most useful for various conditions, and some special notes about each problem.

Arthritis

Your first instinct, when your joints become painful, is to stop moving. Unfortunately, this inactivity usually increases the pain and stiffness over time. During the acute stages, when pain and inflammation are at their worst, you may be able to do only small movements at half capacity, but I urge you to do something, no matter how little, every day; breathing techniques and meditation can always be done, for instance. Do not force yourself to exercise vigorously; err on the side of caution rather than zeal.

Take a warm shower or bath before you exercise to help relax your joints and muscles. Practice the massage techniques (pp. 72–74) before every exercise. Instead of tiring yourself by trying to practice several minutes at a time, practice your exercises throughout the day in small increments. As you go through your Complete Relaxation Procedure (pp. 133–138), visualize your joints and muscles relaxing and the inflammation receding.

Watching your diet can sometimes help arthritis as well. Read p. 160 in the Diet and Nutrition chapter for some specific suggestions.

"Yoga helped me quite a bit. I have arthritis in my hips, legs, and hands. It's just stiff to move, you know. By doing this Yoga exercise, it

helps me get limbered up, and I can bend over more. I can even walk a little better, without so much pain."

—Jim Chesser (age 77)

Asthma and Breathing Disorders

The compression and stretching exercises of Easy Does It Yoga, particularly those that stretch the rib cage, can help relax the respiratory system and prevent or reduce the severity of attacks. Practice the following exercises every day: Frog Pose (p. 76), Side Stretch (p. 77), Arm Reach (p. 65), Arm Swing (p. 70), Knee Squeeze (seated, p. 82, and lying down, p. 116), Cobra Pose (p. 122), and Complete Breath (p. 58).

Poor stress-coping skills can sometimes bring on an asthma attack, because one of the reactions to stress is constricted breathing. The feeling during an attack of not being able to breathe then increases the fear reaction, which is even more stressful. Practice your breathing and meditation techniques every day as a way to help break the cycle by reducing anxiety and fear.

"Back in 1980 I was diagnosed with emphysema and asthma. Fortunately for me I had started to practice Yoga, and any time I had difficulty breathing I would resort to the Easy Does It Yoga exercises. I was able to do these with very little restriction. I feel that the breathing exercises are especially helpful for me. In the past nineteen years my doctor has not had to increase my medication. In fact, I have gradually reduced the amount of prescription medication I take and continue to be in good health."

—Corrine Goodman (age 60)

Back Pain

"Oh, my aching back!" is a common refrain heard from adults of all ages; however, evidence from a study of three thousand back pain cases showed that 83 percent of the patients had no pathological disorder. The pain was due to stiff, weak postural muscles. Tension and physical inactivity were contributing factors in many of their disabilities.

First, consult your doctor to determine if there is a medical reason for the pain, such as a herniated disk. With your doctor's permission, you may begin some limited movements that will help strengthen your back muscles, relieve tension in the lower back, strengthen abdominal muscles, prevent stiffness, and improve circulation to the affected area. At first, do every movement at half capacity; never exercise to the point of pain. Be sure to breathe correctly for every exercise. Do your breathing and meditation techniques every day to help you relax.

Some exercises that may help are the Sun Pose Stretch (p. 110), and the Easy Alternate Sun Pose (p. 112), the Easy Cobra Lift (p. 121), the Knee Squeezes (seated, p. 82, and lying down, p. 116), the Easy Bridge (p. 118), the Alternate Toe Touch (p. 119), and the Back Strengtheners (p. 122). The first three exercises listed above must be done on the floor; the others may be done in bed.

"I began practicing Yoga years ago because I had a severe back problem. I knew I couldn't do all of the Yoga exercises so the teacher helped me modify them with the Easy Does It Yoga program. Little by little I was able to increase my flexibility and strengthen my back."

—Joan Blair (age 65)

Chronic Pain

A common response to pain is to tighten the muscles around the painful area, often making the pain worse instead of better. Yoga helps you relax your muscles at will and also stimulates your body to produce more of the brain chemicals that cause feelings of well-being, so you feel less pain overall. Some students have told me that they use their breathing techniques to help them relax and to distract themselves when they undergo uncomfortable medical or dental procedures.

Try to practice a small daily routine of at least three exercises, a few repetitions of Complete Breath, and at least 10 minutes of meditation. Choose exercises that you enjoy doing and that do not cause additional pain. Throughout the day, practice Easy Does It Yoga techniques whenever you think about it, to keep yourself from becoming stiff and inactive.

"Before this Yoga I didn't know anything about rubbing and stretching and trying to get relief. Just moving my old bones I'd get to crying and crying. These exercises help get some pains out of there, though. They do me good."

—Annie Mae Johnson (age 63)

Circulatory Problems (Heart Disease/Hypertension)

Exercise helps to maintain coronary artery circulation and the flexibility of the large arteries. Exercise improves blood circulation, which is important for bringing nutrients to all parts of the body and removing waste products.

Remember to obtain your doctor's permission and move slowly in all exercises. If you have a pacemaker, you may be advised not to raise your arms above shoulder height. High blood pressure may cause a throbbing or pounding in your head when you bend your head below the level of your heart. If this causes dizziness or discomfort, bend only halfway forward, and practice the supported versions of exercises until you get stronger.

Excessive or prolonged reactions to stress can put unnecessary strain on your heart and circulatory system, and Yoga techniques can help you cope more effectively. Practice the Complete Breath (p. 58) several times a day, especially when you notice yourself remaining tense, anxious, or irritable. When you are concentrating on your breathing, you won't be able to pay attention to stressful thoughts and feelings.

Use the relaxation procedure (pp. 133–138) to help you sleep at night. If much of your day is spent at a desk, practice some simple exercises throughout the day to keep your upper back and neck from becoming tight and fatigued.

See the Diet and Nutrition chapter for information on the role of a proper diet in improving a circulatory problem.

"I started Yoga shortly after having heart surgery seven years ago. In meditation I think of my heart as 'bright red and strong' and I think of my silvery lungs. This imagery not only serves to relax me during meditation, but also rejuvenates my feelings of health."

—Dan Ticktin (age 42)

Constipation

The most prevalent digestive problem in older adults, constipation usually results from a combination of an inactive lifestyle and a diet lacking in fiber (roughage). See p. 161 in the Diet and Nutrition chapter to find out how to get more fiber in your diet, and practice your Easy Does It Yoga exercises every day. Exercises that compress the abdominal area, such as the Standing Knee Squeeze (p. 100) and the Easy Cobra Lift (p. 121), will encourage your digestive organs to function normally.

"It's the knee lifts that helped me the most. I know my Yoga does me good because my knee has always bothered me. I have arthritis in my knee, but it's much better now. I haven't been having the pains very much. In fact, I haven't had much pain all this week, and none last week."

—Agnes Barton (age 64)

Depression

The most important way to counteract depression is to force yourself to move every day. In a depressive episode, you want to stop moving, but this will only perpetuate your depression. If you cannot face the idea of doing a full routine of exercises, do one at a time every hour throughout the day. Do the same with your breathing exercises. Once every hour, breathe deeply three times using either the Complete Breath (p. 58), the Belly Breath (p. 57), or the Humming Breath (p. 60).

Your appetite may be diminished, but it is also important to keep yourself well nourished. Enlist the help of a friend to remind you to eat or to share a treat now and then. Make mealtimes pleasant and appealing by adding something special, such as watching a favorite videotape, taking food on a tray to eat on your porch or in the backyard, or lighting candles.

Diabetes

Diabetics are at risk for circulatory problems, especially in the extremities. Yoga can help improve circulation. Practice the exercises that use your entire body, such as the Seated Full Bend Breath (p. 86), the Full Bend Twist (p. 88), the Simple Alternate Triangle (p. 104), and the Knee Squeezes (seated, p. 82, and lying down, p. 116). Practice the Complete Breath every day to improve your concentration and willpower, especially if you are trying to lose weight.

A nutritious diet is extremely important for diabetics. See p. 162 in the Diet and Nutrition chapter for more information.

Incontinence

Incontinence is not an inevitable result of aging, as many people believe, but simply a weakening of certain muscles through disuse. A daily routine of Easy Does It Yoga exercise, breathing, and meditation can rebuild this muscle strength very quickly. Include in your daily routine the technique shown on p. 129 to strengthen your muscles and correct the problem. This technique can be done in bed; for best results, practice it twice daily at least, and add repetitions any time you are at rest during the day.

Obesity

If you are severely overweight, you are probably very inactive as well. Start with a small daily routine that you know you can stick to: Commit to three exercises of your choice, three Complete Breath cycles, and a few minutes of relaxation. Add more exercises and lengthen the time you spend breathing and relaxing whenever you like. The longer you maintain the commitment to daily practice, the more you will benefit.

Take care not to rush into any strenuous exercises, and be careful not to strain the joints of your hips, knees, and ankles, which may be especially weak. Practice breathing techniques every day; this will help boost your concentration and willpower. Weight loss is slow but steady with attention to diet and Easy Does It Yoga exercise.

Read the Diet and Nutrition chapter for advice on planning a nutritious diet that will help you lose weight and stay healthy.

Osteoporosis

Osteoporosis (brittle bones) is a major health problem that begins as early as ages thirty to thirty-five and affects about 25 million Americans, 80 percent of them women. Although the primary cause of osteoporosis is a lack of dietary calcium in the years up to age thirty when bones are still growing, inactivity also contributes to this disorder, which causes the bones to become so weak that they break easily.

A regular program of strength training and weight-bearing exercise can help improve bone density. Any of the standing exercises of Easy Does It Yoga (pp. 92–105) will complement other weight-bearing exercises recommended by your physician. Also practice the Leg and Arm Strengtheners described as warm-ups to the floor exercises (p. 107).

Adding calcium to your diet now will also help. Nonfat or low-fat dairy products (milk and yogurt are the best), tofu, and greens such as kale and spinach are good sources of calcium. In order to get as much calcium as is generally recommended (1,500 mg daily for women), you may need to supplement your diet (consult your doctor or a nutritionist for advice). Read pp. 164–165 in the Diet and Nutrition chapter for more information.

Severely Limited Movement or Paralysis

My teacher, Rama, told me that even thinking about performing a Yoga exercise would have a beneficial effect. He advised me to do this once long ago when I had broken my back and was in too much pain to practice the Yoga exercises daily. I am fully recovered now, and I always recommend this technique to persons who are temporarily limited in their movement. Modern science seems to agree with this advice; studies have shown that when you think about moving a part of your body, electrical impulses to that area actually increase.

If you are completely paralyzed, you can definitely practice the breathing and meditation every day, and you should also do some exercises in your mind. Read the instructions, then close your eyes and imagine yourself doing the exercise exactly as instructed. Be sure to breathe correctly as well. Try to imagine your body working perfectly as you concentrate.

If you are partially paralyzed, adapt the exercises for yourself so that you are making full use of your functioning limbs; at the same time, imagine that your entire body is functioning perfectly as you do the exercise. Bring the strength of your concentration to the injured spot.

Substance Abuse Recovery

Addiction makes you forget the strength of your own resources; Yoga helps you remember who you are and what you are capable of doing. As a general rule, you'll find that as you become stronger and healthier, your body will naturally tend to reject things that will harm it, making it easier to resist relapse. Often a factor in addiction is a lack of appropriate stress-coping skills. Regular practice of Yoga techniques will help you respond to the stresses in your life more effectively.

Recovery from addiction to cigarettes, alcohol, prescription drugs, or other substances need not be painful. During the initial detox period, you should make every attempt to give your body and mind the most loving care by eating healthy, balanced meals that are rich in protein and vitamins B and C (see the Diet and Nutrition chapter). Drink plenty of water, get plenty of rest, and avoid upsetting or stressful situations if you can.

After the detox period, your primary focus should be on gaining strength and building healthy lifestyle habits to replace the addicting ones. Easy Does It Yoga provides some simple movements and techniques that can be done any time of day to increase your activity levels gradually. Any of the chair exercises, for example, can be done at your desk or while you watch television, and you can practice the Complete Breath any time you remember to try it. Make a commitment to practice a few minutes of Easy Does It Yoga exercise, breathing, and meditation every day. You will find that Yoga acts as a natural stimulant by increasing your energy level, making it easier to keep your commitment to daily practice. The breathing techniques will increase your concentration and willpower, and regular meditation practice will increase your sense of self-worth.

If your addiction was to sleeping aids, try practicing a few minutes of breathing exercises in bed, followed by the Complete Relaxation Procedure (see p. 133), for a natural calming effect that will help you sleep without drugs.

If you are trying to stop smoking, counteract the urge for a cigarette by doing a few Complete Breaths or a few Easy Does It Yoga exercises. The feeling of well-being that results will likely drown out the addictive urge.

YOUR SUPPORT SYSTEM

Easy Does It Yoga gives you a full range of healthy lifestyle choices to support you during stressful times—convalescence, major life changes, or simply when you deal with the many day-to-day frustrations that often add up to stressful feelings. Set aside some time each day for Yoga, and you will soon see how that daily commitment builds a constant feeling of steadiness and well-being that supports you in life like the waters of a calm lake.

A POSITIVE ATTITUDE

A creative, supportive, and friendly attitude toward your body and mind will bring you the best and fastest results in Easy Does It Yoga. Be optimistic about your capabilities. Gently stretch your limitations and be appreciative of the opportunity to learn how to become healthier and more energetic.

A doctor once told Rama, "You aren't getting any younger, you know. You shouldn't walk so fast. Slow down!" Rama replied, "Young man, when I'm dead and let go of this body, maybe then it will slow down; until then it will remain active—along with me!"

Look on your practice of Easy Does It Yoga as a new, enjoyable way to live the life you want and become the person you want to be. Set up your routine so that you really enjoy it and look forward to it. You will love the quick results.

CHAPTER 3

Six Weeks with Easy Does It Yoga

"I have had a muscle problem for over twenty-five years, which has kept me from doing many things, even household chores. My lower back and shoulders have been in constant pain, and my muscles ached all over and were sore to the touch. I never had a sense of 'well-being'—in fact, most days I felt really bad. I always felt inside that exercise might help, but not one doctor ever encouraged me. In fact, most even discouraged me. I have now been practicing Easy Does It Yoga for over three months, and the change is remarkable. I am no longer afraid to move for fear of muscle spasms, and my muscles feel much stronger. The pain in my lower back is completely gone, and the pain between my shoulders only returns if I overdo with my arms. This also is getting better. The pain used to be constant, nagging, and often very severe. But now, it's relieved. I'm much more flexible."

—Charlotte Shade (age 60)

Before heading into the chapters that teach you the Easy Does It Yoga techniques, you may wish to learn how to combine the techniques into a daily routine. This chapter gives a suggested six-week outline to guide you on your way to a healthier, happier life. You won't have time every day to practice every technique in this book; use these outlines to establish yourself in a basic routine of essential movements, then add any other techniques you wish.

The exercises listed for each week will take 10 to 20 minutes to complete. Each list begins with a few warm-up exercises, then progresses to chair exercises, standing exercises, and eventually floor exercises. Practice the techniques in the order presented, and, as mentioned in the Getting Started chapter, practice every day for best results.

If you are coping with chronic health problems, have special limitations, or are more active, modify the routine as needed to give yourself a challenge but not wear yourself out. The suggested exercises become more difficult each week; you can choose among them to create a routine that you like to do and that is not too strenuous for you.

Be sure to familiarize yourself with all the cautions and hints discussed in the Getting Started chapter before you begin. Rest frequently between exercises, and massage your joints often (see pp. 72–74).

WEEK ONE

Warm-up Exercises

    Shoulder Roll, p. 67

    Arm Reach, p. 65

    Elbow Roll and Elbow Touch, p. 66

Seated Exercises

    Seated Leg Lift and Foot Flaps, p. 80

    Massage, p. 72

    Seated Knee Squeeze, p. 82

    Folded Pose, p. 84

Standing Exercises

    Strut, p. 92

    Ankle Strengtheners, p. 93

    Lazy Knee Bends, p. 107

    Tip-Toe Balance, p. 96

    Standing Reach, p. 94

Breathing

    Belly Breath, p. 57 (5–10 repetitions)

Meditation

    10 minutes lying down (floor or bed)

Nutrition

    Read chapter 9 and begin to read labels when you go grocery shopping. Carefully check your purchases for nutritional value. Don't buy chemicals; spend your money on food.

Philosophy

    Read chapter 10 and study the "Five Ways to Increase Personal Growth." Make a real attempt this week to live in the present.

WEEK TWO

Warm-up Exercises

    Shoulder Roll, p. 67

    Arm Reach, p. 65

    Elbow Roll and Elbow Touch, p. 66

    Arm Circles, p. 69

    Arm Swing, p. 70

    Neck Stretches, p. 70

Seated Exercises

    Throat Tightener, p. 68

    Facial Exercises, p. 75

    Seated Leg Lift and Foot Flaps, p. 80

    Massage, p. 72

    Seated Knee Squeeze, p. 82

    Folded Pose, p. 84

    Elbow to Knee, p. 89

    Seated Full Bend Breath, p. 86

Standing Exercises
    Strut, p. 92
    Ankle Strengtheners, p. 93
    Lazy Knee Bends, p. 107
    Tip-Toe Balance, p. 96
    Standing Leg Lifts, p. 99
    Leg and Arm Strengtheners, p. 107
Breathing
    Belly Breath, p. 57 (5–10 repetitions)
    Complete Breath, p. 58 (5–10 repetitions)
Meditation
    10–15 minutes lying down (bed or floor)
Nutrition
    Make a list of everything you eat this week. At the end
    of the week, compare your list to the menu suggestions on
    pp. 153–156.
Philosophy
    Pick one of the ethical guidelines described on p. 170 and
    concentrate on following it this week. Keep a journal of
    your experiences and thoughts if you wish. This can be
    fun to share with a friend.

WEEK THREE
Warm-up Exercises
    Shoulder Roll, p. 67
    Arm Reach, p. 65
    Elbow Roll and Elbow Touch, p. 66
    Arm Circles, p. 69
    Arm Swing, p. 70
    Neck Stretches, p. 70
Seated Exercises
    Eye Exercises, p. 132
    Seated Leg Lift and Foot Flaps, p. 80
    Massage, p. 72
    Full Bend Twist, p. 88
    Seated Knee Squeeze, p. 82
    Folded Pose, p. 84
    Shoulder to Knee, p. 90
    Seated Full Bend Breath, p. 86
Standing Exercises
    Strut, p. 92
    Ankle Strengtheners, p. 93
    Lazy Knee Bends, p. 107
    Tip-Toe Balance, p. 96
    Standing Leg Lifts, p. 99
    Rear Arm Lift, p. 101

Gentle Full Bends, p. 97
Standing Knee Squeeze, p. 100
Breathing
Complete Breath, p. 58 (5–10 repetitions)
Relaxing Breath, p. 60 (in bed or on the floor)
Meditation
15–20 minutes lying down (bed or floor)
Nutrition

If last week's comparison showed you that you were eating more "junk" and less real food, start this week and substitute a more healthy food. For instance, if you are drinking a lot of coffee every day, make every cup half skim milk; or just drink less coffee and drink more water and fruit juice instead.

Philosophy

Try forming a study group with a few of your friends and pick one of the books on the reading list to read and discuss together. Or just read the book yourself, copying out sentences or paragraphs that strike you and posting them on your refrigerator, where you can see and think about them every day.

WEEK FOUR
Warm-up Exercises
Shoulder Roll, p. 67
Arm Reach, p. 65
Elbow Roll and Elbow Touch, p. 66
Arm Circles, p. 69
Arm Swing, p. 70
Neck Stretches, p. 70
Seated Exercises
Eye Exercises, p. 132
The Lion, p. 76
Frog Pose, p. 76
Side Stretch, p. 77
Full Bend Twist, p. 88
Seated Knee Squeeze, p. 82
Massage, p. 72
Folded Pose, p. 84
Standing Exercises
Strut, p. 92
Ankle Strengtheners, p. 93
Lazy Knee Bends, p. 107
Tip-Toe Balance, p. 96
Standing Leg Lifts, p. 99
Rear Arm Lift, p. 101

Gentle Full Bends, p. 97
Standing Knee Squeeze, p. 100
Floor Exercises
Getting Down on the Floor, p. 108
Gentle Twist, p. 113
Foot Flap, p. 81
Seated Sun Pose, p. 111
Breathing
Complete Breath, p. 58 (5–10 repetitions)
Humming Breath, p. 60 (3–5 repetitions)
Meditation
15–20 minutes, lying down (bed or floor)
Nutrition

This week, concentrate on your snacking habits. Substitute healthy foods such as raw vegetables, fruit, or low-fat pretzels for candy or chips. Skim milk, yogurt, or cottage cheese are also good as snacks in themselves, or they can be made into delicious dips for raw vegetables, fruit, or pretzels.

Philosophy

Seek out new and challenging relationships. Take a course at a local school, or join a club, or become more involved in a church or synagogue. Ask a friend to join your Yoga program and have fun comparing results.

WEEK FIVE
Warm-up Exercises
Shoulder Roll, p. 67
Arm Reach, p. 65
Elbow Roll and Elbow Touch, p. 66
Arm Circles, p. 69
Arm Swing, p. 70
Neck Stretches, p. 70
Seated Exercises
Eye Exercises, p. 132
The Lion, p. 76
Frog Pose, p. 76
Side Stretch, p. 77
Seated Twist, p. 79
Laughing Bicycle, p. 83
Seated Knee Squeeze, p. 82
Massage, p. 72
Folded Pose, p. 84
Standing Exercises
Tree Pose, p. 102
Simple Alternate Triangle, p. 104

Lazy Knee Bends, p. 107
Standing Leg Lifts, p. 99
Rear Arm Lift, p. 101
Gentle Full Bends, p. 97

Floor Exercises
Getting Down on the Floor, p. 108
Gentle Twist, p. 113
Foot Flap, p. 81
Seated Sun Pose, p. 111
Easy Alternate Sun Pose, p. 112
Knee Squeeze, p. 116
Easy Bridge, p. 118
Easy Cobra Lift, p. 121
All-Fours Lift, p. 124

Breathing
Complete Breath, p. 58 (5–10 repetitions)
Humming Breath, p. 60 (3–5 repetitions)
Stomach Lift, p. 61

Meditation
If you wish, try a seated meditation this week. Review the instructions on p. 134 for relaxing in a seated position.

Nutrition
Concentrate on reducing your sugar intake this week. Rather than substituting "sugar-free" chemicals, try to change your tastes to natural foods such as fruit, or substitute a small amount of honey. Try a new brand of breakfast cereal that has less added sugar.

Philosophy
Set realistic daily, weekly, or yearly goals and put the steps in motion to achieve them. Decide what you really want out of life and plan how to achieve it.

WEEK SIX
Warm-up Exercises
Shoulder Roll, p. 67
Arm Reach, p. 65
Elbow Touch, p. 66
Arm Circles, p. 69
Arm Swing, p. 70
Neck Stretches, p. 70

Seated Exercises
Eye Exercises, p. 132
The Lion, p. 76
Frog Pose, p. 76
Side Stretch, p. 77

Seated Twist, p. 79
Massage, p. 72
Laughing Bicycle, p. 83

Standing Exercises

Gentle Full Bends, p. 97
Tree Pose, p. 102
Simple Alternate Triangle, p. 104
Rear Leg Lifts and Super Balance Pose, p. 103
Rear Arm Lift, p. 101

Floor Exercises

Getting Down on the Floor, p. 108
Spine Twist, p. 114
Foot Flap, p. 81
Seated Sun Pose, p. 111
Alternate Tortoise Stretch, p. 115
All-Fours Lift, p. 124
Baby Pose, p. 125
Knee Squeeze, p. 116
Alternate Toe Touch, p. 119
Easy Bridge, p. 118
Lower Back Stretch, p. 120
Easy Cobra Lift, p. 121
Back Strengtheners, p. 122

Breathing

Complete Breath, p. 58 (5–10 repetitions)
Humming Breath, p. 60 (3–5 repetitions)
Stomach Lift, p. 61 (3 repetitions)

Meditation

15–20 minutes, seated or lying down

Nutrition

If you are trying to lose weight, start by shifting the time of day that you eat your biggest meal. As the saying goes, "Eat breakfast like a king, lunch like a prince, and supper like a pauper." If you are disciplined enough to eat the right foods more often, an even better plan is to eat six small meals throughout the day rather than three large ones.

Philosophy

Pick another of the ethical guidelines discussed on p. 170 and try to put it into practice in everyday life. Choose a different one every week and see what a difference it makes in your outlook.

"I work in a hospital and often must position patients that have limited movement. Although I have been trained to lift and position patients

and I always use another person to help, at least once a month I used to strain my back. Since I started doing my daily Yoga stretches, I have not hurt my back in over three years."

—Yvonne Wolfe (age 47)

WHEELCHAIR AND BED ROUTINES

Wheelchair Routine

Your chair should be locked in place, and your feet should be firmly supported while you do these exercises. Try to do the Bed Routine exercises every day as well to help prevent sores, improve circulation, and keep your joints and muscles from becoming stiff and weak. You may feel insecure about attempting forward-bending exercises, especially if your legs are weak. Never force yourself to do anything that feels uncomfortable; do the exercise bending only halfway forward, or ask a friend or family member to stand near you in case you lose your balance. Remember that you can practice these techniques any time of day to increase the benefits.

The weekly outlines are designed to build strength and flexibility and to provide variety. You should notice an increase in self-confidence and a greater feeling of connection with your body movements as you progress through this four-week outline.

WEEK ONE
Belly Breath, p. 57
Shoulder Roll, p. 67
Elbow Roll, p. 66
Arm Reach, p. 65
Neck Stretches, p. 70
Arm Circles, p. 69
Foot Flap and Ankle Rotation, p. 81
Seated Leg Lift, p. 80
Seated Full Bend Breath, p. 86
Massage, p. 72
Seated Knee Squeeze, p. 82
Frog Pose, p. 76
Complete Relaxation Procedure, p. 133

WEEK TWO
Complete Breath, p. 58
Shoulder Roll, p. 67
Elbow Roll, p. 66
Arm Reach, p. 65

Facial Exercises, p. 75
Throat Tightener, p. 68
Eye Exercises, p. 132
Arm Swing, p. 70
Neck Stretches, p. 70
Arm Circles, p. 69
Side Stretch, p. 77
Foot Flap and Ankle Rotation, p. 81
Seated Leg Lift, p. 80
Seated Full Bend Breath, p. 86
Massage, p. 72
Full Bend Twist, p. 88
The Lion, p. 76
Frog Pose, p. 76
Seated Knee Squeeze, p. 82
Elbow to Knee, p. 89
Folded Pose, p. 84
Seated Twist, p. 79
Laughing Bicycle, p. 83
Humming Breath, p. 60
Complete Relaxation Procedure, p. 133

Bed Routine

If you can sit on the edge of the bed with your feet on the floor, you may add some of the chair exercises to your routine. Do not attempt any forward-bending seated exercises unless your feet are firmly supported on the floor. If you are unsure about your balance, ask a friend or family member to stand close to you while you try the forward-bending poses, or keep a chair that won't slip in front of you in case you need extra support. Some excellent techniques to try are the Seated Leg Lift (p. 80), the Seated Knee Squeeze (p. 82), and the Seated Twist (p. 79). Also, many of the upper-body exercises can be done lying on your side, alternating sides so that one arm works at a time. Practice the techniques any time of day to increase the benefits.

WEEK ONE
Belly Breath, p. 57
Shoulder Roll, p. 67
Elbow Roll, p. 66
Arm Reach, p. 65
Arm Swing, p. 70
Neck Stretches, p. 70
Foot Flap and Ankle Rotation, p. 81
Knee Squeeze, p. 116

Alternate Toe Touch, p. 119
Massage, p. 72
Easy Bridge, p. 118
Complete Relaxation Procedure, p. 133

WEEK TWO
Complete Breath, p. 58
Shoulder Roll, p. 67
Elbow Roll, p. 66
Arm Reach, p. 65
Arm Swing, p. 70
Neck Stretches, p. 70
Facial Exercises, p. 75
Throat Tightener, p. 68
Foot Flap and Ankle Rotation, p. 81
Knee Squeeze, p. 116
Alternate Toe Touch, p. 119
Laughing Bicycle, p. 83
Massage, p. 72
Easy Bridge, p. 118
Incontinence Relief, p. 129
Complete Relaxation Procedure, p. 133

WEEK THREE
Complete Breath, p. 58
Shoulder Roll, p. 67
Elbow Roll, p. 66
Arm Reach, p. 65
Arm Swing, p. 70
Neck Stretches, p. 70
Facial Exercises, p. 75
Throat Tightener, p. 68
Foot Flap and Ankle Rotation, p. 81
Knee Squeeze, p. 116
Alternate Toe Touch, p. 119
Lower Back Stretch, p. 120
Laughing Bicycle, p. 83
Massage, p. 72
Easy Bridge, p. 118
Incontinence Relief, p. 129
Humming Breath, p. 60
Complete Relaxation Procedure, p. 133

WEEK FOUR
Complete Breath, p. 58
Shoulder Roll, p. 67

"I have more energy and I am actually participating in life again, and it's great. I know I've got to be regular in my routine to maintain and improve my progress, but it's really wonderful to know that by doing this Easy Does It Yoga, I have a chance to feel better than I have in years. I find life exciting again and good. And my husband thinks I'm much more fun to be with."

—Charlotte Shade (age 60)

TECHNIQUES GROUPED BY BENEFITS

Once you have established a basic routine for yourself, either by following the weekly outlines presented earlier in this chapter or by creating your own routine, you will begin to understand how the different exercises affect you physically. For instance, you may notice that when you practice the Frog Pose, your back doesn't feel so stiff. In this section, you will find the exercises and other techniques listed in categories according to how they affect your body. Use these lists to add a few extra exercises to your routine when you want to help yourself in a specific way. For instance, you may wake up one morning feeling depressed. Add the techniques listed as Energizers to your daily routine to help yourself feel better.

Face, Neck, Shoulders, Upper Back
Chair

Arm Reach, p. 65
Shoulder Roll, p. 67
Throat Tightener, p. 68
Arm Swing, p. 70

Improved Digestion
Chair
>Seated Knee Squeeze, p. 82
>Folded Pose, p. 84
>Elbow to Knee, p. 89
>Shoulder to Knee, p. 90
>Seated Twist, p. 79
>Seated Full Bend Breath, p. 86
>Full Bend Twist, p. 88

Standing
>Gentle Full Bends, p. 97
>Standing Knee Squeeze, p. 100

Floor
>Knee Squeeze, p. 116
>Sun Pose Stretch, p. 110
>Seated Sun Pose, p. 111
>Gentle Twist, p. 113
>Stomach Lift, p. 61

ENERGIZERS

Energizers are any techniques that improve oxygenation by expanding the chest wall, increase upper body circulation, bring a fresh blood supply to the head, and/or stretch and contract postural muscles. Use these techniques when you are feeling depressed, recovering from jet lag, or facing a difficult day ahead. These techniques will help you look and feel your best; they will bring a brightness into your face and a lightness into your carriage.

>Elbow Roll, p. 66
>Shoulder Roll, p. 67
>Frog Pose, p. 76
>Folded Pose, p. 84
>Gentle Full Bends, p. 97
>Arm Reach, p. 65
>Laughing Bicycle, p. 83
>Arm Swing, p. 70

RELAXERS

Relaxers are any techniques that release tension in the stomach and breathing muscles, release facial tension, compress the abdomen, and/or focus attention inward on the breath process or on the relaxation process. Use them to calm yourself after a stressful encounter, to help you sleep better, or to reduce anxiety.

CHAPTER 4

How to Start Breathing Better

"I used to get so tense. Sometimes I get really angry, especially if I'm around people who are very trying. My breathing has helped me tolerate them a lot better. I can be more patient with them. Now, when I get angry, I just take a few deep, slow breaths. I come out of that angry feeling and just relax. My whole tone changes, and I can talk to them real close, just real gentle. I can just handle situations like that better now because of my breathing."

—Jeanne Hrovat (age 66)

Almost every Yoga exercise includes a specific breath pattern, which is an essential part of making the exercise work for you. Note also that each technique usually begins with three Complete Breaths. This focuses your attention on the breath, which will help to insure that you keep breathing throughout the exercise.

If you have become very inactive due to age or illness, you are probably breathing less deeply than you used to; this contributes to feelings of lethargy and weakness which, in turn, contribute to further inactivity. Unless your muscles are exercised, they lose their elasticity at an alarming rate—and this includes the muscles that you use for breathing, such as your diaphragm and the muscles between your ribs. People who are inactive also usually have poor posture and weak back and stomach muscles, which creates a chronic slouch that also inhibits breathing. This combination of inactivity, slouching, and muscle stiffness causes your body and brain to get much less oxygen than they should, which often results in depression. The natural process of aging also affects the efficiency of your breath—but this inefficiency can be reversed.

In this chapter you will learn how to breathe more completely, using the important diaphragm muscle as well as the many other muscles that your body needs to use for breathing. This technique trains your lungs to fill and empty more fully, allowing more oxygen in and pushing more waste products out. Most students observe that after practicing this technique for some time, they find themselves breathing more deeply at other times of the day as well, because they are more conscious of their breath patterns.

BENEFITS OF BETTER BREATHING

When you have learned how to breathe more effectively, you will feel more alert, energetic, and alive. Training yourself to breathe deeply and completely will also improve your concentration, memory, and stamina.

Many students have told me that they use their deep breathing exercises to help relieve anxiety, anger, fear, or other strong feelings associated with stress. Every one of us faces stressful situations such as family problems, living on a fixed income or with other financial pressures, medical or dental problems, and loneliness. You will discover that your breath is closely related to emotion. Think for a moment about what happens to your breath when you are depressed, angry, afraid, or excited. When you feel depressed, for instance, you find yourself sighing a lot, and your breath becomes slow and shallow. When you are afraid or angry, on the other hand, your breath often speeds up. If you practice breathing techniques regularly, you will find that keeping your breath deeper and more regular will help you to change your mood and feel happier and more in control.

Breathing techniques can be extremely helpful in pain management and sleeping problems as well. If you must undergo uncomfortable medical procedures, or if you suffer from chronic pain, try using the breathing techniques to relax your body and mind and take your mind off the discomfort. A greater regular supply of oxygen will result in more restful sleeping patterns.

"It's made me more alert. It seems like I get more air, more energy, and everybody's remarking about how much more alert I seem."
—Jeanne Hrovat (age 66)

OTHER FACTORS THAT AFFECT BREATHING

Smoking

If you smoke, now is a good time to stop! Not only does smoking contribute to heart disease and cancer, it also inhibits breathing. Longtime smokers often experience shortness of breath and a chronic cough that keeps them from breathing deeply. Bronchitis and emphysema are two serious breathing-related diseases that result from smoking. It's never too late to benefit from giving up tobacco. To help yourself quit, practice breathing techniques several times a day to strengthen your lungs and reduce anxiety.

Excess Weight

Being overweight puts a strain on your lungs as well as your heart. Recent surveys show that almost half of the American population is overweight. Although it is probably natural to gain a little weight as we grow older, it is easy to gain too much if you are inactive and lack the energy to change your lifestyle. Many people also eat as a nervous habit, out of fear or anxiety, and often eat less nutritious foods. Breathing techniques help to improve concentration, energy, and willpower, making it easier to change the lifestyle habits that are keeping those extra pounds on.

"I do the breathing exercises quite a bit, sometimes even in church. Both my wife's and my breathing have improved a lot."

—John Sleda (age 75)

HOW TO START BREATHING BETTER

There are several important aspects to learning how to breathe better:

Correct Posture

It's very important to keep your back straight during breathing exercises. Practice the techniques sitting in a straight chair, not leaning against the chair back. (After you have learned the technique, you can practice it anytime, anywhere.) The position will be more comfortable if there is a slight downward slant from your hips to your knees; try sitting on the edge of the chair and tucking your toes under slightly to achieve this position. If you tend to slouch due to weak muscles, you can practice the breathing with your chair pushed sideways against a wall (see photo). Sit sideways in the chair with hips and shoulders touching the wall; this will prevent your back from slouching forward during the exhalation.

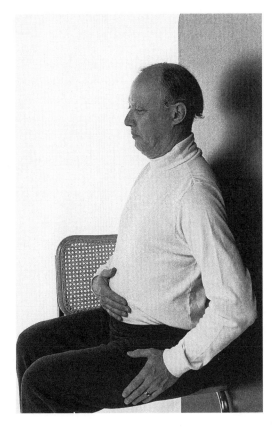

You can also practice breathing techniques while lying flat in bed or on the floor, with knees bent (see Relaxing Breath, p. 60). Don't put a pillow under your head or neck (unless medically necessary).

If you have access to a pool, you may wish to try practicing your breathing exercises sitting on a step in the pool so that your stomach and part of your chest are submerged. This will increase the resistance and strengthen your breathing muscles considerably.

Always Breathe Through Your Nose

Many people approach any exercise class with the idea of breathing out through pursed lips, as is done in many calisthenic-type exercise programs. Many older people have developed the habit of breathing through their mouth, which seems to bring them more oxygen. In Yoga, always breathe in *and* out through your nose (unless you have a specific airway problem and your doctor has told you to breathe out through your mouth). Breathing through the nose affects the nervous system differently from mouth breathing. It allows for a slower and more deliberate inhalation and exhalation, and it will improve your concentration and stamina. With practice, you will experience just as much oxygen intake as with mouth breathing.

Sometimes you will find one or the other nostril blocked. If blowing your nose gently does not clear it, try the following simple technique: If your right nostril is blocked, make a fist with your right hand. Place the fist in your left armpit and lower your left arm over it, which will exert some pressure on your fist and press it into your body. Hold for a minute or two, and soon your right nostril will open so you can breathe freely. Reverse positions for a blockage on the left side.

Use Your Stomach Muscles

To use your diaphragm fully, the belly should go *out* when the breath comes in, and should come *in* when the breath goes out. This is opposite to the way most people have been breathing throughout their lives. Most people breathe from the upper portion of their chest; when they breathe in, they suck their stomach in so that the chest expands more. In the breathing techniques taught in this chapter, your most important task will be to learn how to reverse your usual breathing pattern so you learn to use your diaphragm and belly muscles to breathe as well as your upper chest. This not only helps you breathe better, but also firms your stomach muscles.

Wear Loose Clothing

If you are wearing tight waistbands or any constricting garments, you will have trouble breathing completely. Wear loose, comfortable, warm clothing so you can breathe fully and more comfortably.

Pay Attention to the Sound of the Breath

Notice the steamlike sound of your breath and concentrate on it as you do your breathing techniques. This will help you breathe more slowly and deeply and will also improve your concentration.

> *"I have bronchitis and asthma, and I also have emphysema, which makes it hard to breathe, especially if I get an infection. I can't just give in to these physical limitations. If I don't feel like I'm doing something about it I get depressed and stressed. And believe me, when you feel that each breath may be your last, that's stressful! I have to work hard at breathing. I get short of breath quickly. I even have trouble doing light housework. My Yoga has definitely helped me increase my breath capacity."*
>
> —Dorothy Wild (age 69)

BELLY BREATH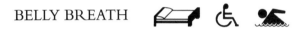

How Will This Exercise Help?

Helps in coping with stress, improves emotional balance, promotes relaxation of the body and mind, strengthens the diaphragm and eyesight, tones the abdominal muscles, and helps to rehabilitate those with chronic lung disease.

Special Notes

Keep your back straight throughout and be careful not to bend forward during exhalation. If you start to feel lightheaded, *do not continue.* Stop and breathe normally until the feeling passes.

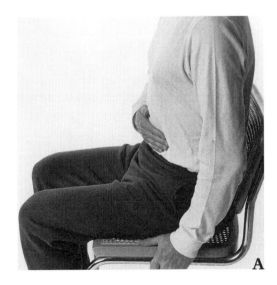

1. Sit up straight and do not lean against the back of your chair. Spread your fingers and hands low on your belly.
2. Slowly breathe in deeply through your nose. (If air is not flowing freely in both nostrils, use the technique on p. 56 to open the blocked side.)
3. As you begin to breathe out, push firmly on your belly in and up, gently forcing the air out with your hands (A).

4. As you start to breathe in, let your belly drop down and out like a balloon being filled with air (B).
5. Repeat Steps 3 and 4 several times, breathing slowly and deeply through your nose. Remember to expand your belly as you breathe in, and contract the belly as you breathe out.

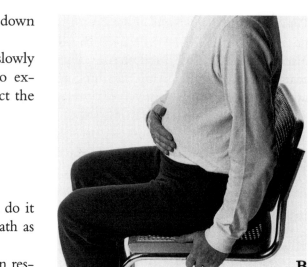

B

Variations

When you have mastered the technique, you can do it without using your hands. Practice the Belly Breath as often during the day as you remember.

Practicing this exercise in a pool will strengthen respiratory muscles due to the increased resistance from the water.

"I have a lot of tension and pressure in my life. When I get real tense and keyed up the deep breathing and meditation really really help."

—Josephine Vidmar (age 70)

COMPLETE BREATH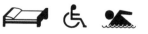

How Will This Exercise Help?

This technique is refreshing, invigorating, and has a calming effect. It helps to relieve depression, boredom, and anxiety. The Complete Breath strengthens and loosens respiratory muscles, improves posture, increases stamina, and tones abdominal muscles.

Special Notes

Remember to check your posture throughout the exercise and keep your back, head, and neck straight. If you tend to slouch forward as you exhale and straighten as you inhale, you will be moving your back muscles more than your breathing muscles.

The first part of this exercise teaches you how to expand your rib cage by raising your arms as you breathe in. In the second part of the exercise, your hands should rest on the hips or legs—never in your lap, because that will constrict your rib cage.

Allow about 10 seconds for each breath (5 seconds inhalation and 5 exhalation). In the Complete Breath, the inhalation and exhalation should be roughly equal in length. Remember always to breathe through your nose, and concentrate on the steamlike sound of the breath.

1. Sit up straight, away from the back of your chair, with your arms at your sides and toes tucked under slightly.
2. Slowly breathe out through your nose, tightening your belly muscles.
3. Start to breathe in, filling and expanding your belly first, as you raise your arms to the sides in a big circle. Continue breathing in, filling your chest all the way up to your shoulders as your arms reach over your head.
4. Start to breathe out, starting from your shoulders and chest, and lowering your arms to your sides in time with your breath. Pull in your belly to get the last of the air out, in the manner of a pumping action.
5. Repeat 5 to 10 times. Rest for at least a minute after the last repetition.
6. Put your hands on your hips or thighs, but keep your arms away from your rib cage so you can breathe deeply.
7. Slowly breathe out through your nose, tightening your belly muscles.
8. Start to breathe in, filling and expanding your belly first, then filling your chest all the way up to your shoulders.
9. Breathe out slowly, letting your shoulders and chest relax first, then pull in your belly to push the last of the air out.
10. Repeat several times, making the inhalation and exhalation roughly equal in length. Rest completely for a few minutes afterward.

Variation

This exercise is also effective when you do it in the pool.

> *"I was terribly short of breath—sometimes I couldn't walk much because of that. Now that I do that long breath, well, it helps. I'm getting around a little better."*
> —Annie Mae Johnson (age 63)

HUMMING BREATH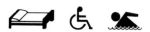

How Will This Exercise Help?

This exercise strengthens breathing muscles and improves concentration when you focus on a steady sound while exhaling. Improves eyesight and memory.

Special Notes

Don't be discouraged if your voice sounds wobbly at first. The point of this exercise is to keep the tone as steady as you can.

1. Sit straight in your chair with hands on your hips. Breathe in and out three times.
2. Breathe in completely, just as in the Complete Breath.
3. Breathe out with an audible "hummmm" sound, making the tone steady and loud until your breath is gone—just like the sound of a bumblebee. Let the sound vibrate in your throat, and keep pushing with your belly muscles so that the sound doesn't trail off at the end. Try to keep the sound steady. Repeat several times.

RELAXING BREATH

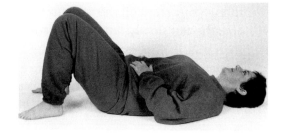

How Will This Exercise Help?

This breathing exercise can be done by anyone in bed or on the floor. In this position, your back is naturally kept straight and you can concentrate on the movement of your belly and chest muscles. This exercise can help with insomnia, and improves eyesight, heart and lung function, and stamina.

Special Notes

Do not put a pillow under your head or neck (unless a medical problem requires it). Your legs will be most comfortable if the toes are pointed slightly in, so that your knees rest together. This is a good technique to do right at the end of your session of floor exercises. Then you can just stretch your legs out and go right into meditation.

1. Lie on your back with your knees bent and feet flat on the floor. Separate your feet several inches and lean your knees against each other. Place your hands on your belly just as in the Belly Breath. Close your eyes.
2. Start to breathe in and out through your nose, just as in the Complete Breath. Your belly will rise up as you inhale and drop down as you exhale. Focus your attention on the sound and feeling of the breath and try to ignore any other sounds or thoughts. Feel yourself relaxing more each time you exhale. Try to make the inhalation and exhalation approximately the same length. Continue breathing for 1–3 minutes.

"I would just lie in bed at night and my breath just seemed so shallow that it made it difficult to fall asleep. It wasn't until I started this Yoga that I ever learned how to breathe deeply."

—Josephine Vidmar (age 70)

STOMACH LIFT

How Will This Exercise Help?

Strengthens abdominal and back muscles, limbers spine, improves breathing and digestion, and also helps prevent incontinence. Improves sexual function.

Special Notes

If you have painful or arthritic knees, do this exercise on a foam mat or a soft blanket; the exercise can also be done on a firm bed. If you have disk problems in your neck, be careful not to strain.

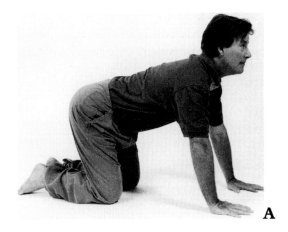

1. Start on your hands and knees, with your back and neck in a straight line. Breathe in and out three times through your nose.
2. Breathe out completely, then breathe in as you arch your back and look up toward the ceiling (A). Hold your breath in for a count of three.

A

3. Breathe out as you round your back, tuck your chin toward your chest, and pull in and up on your stomach muscles (B). Hold your breath out for a count of three.
4. Breathe in and relax. Rest for several seconds, then repeat twice more.

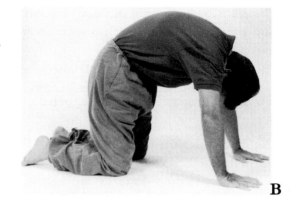

B

Variations

If you are unable to put weight on your knees, you can do this exercise in a standing position: Start by separating your feet several inches, bending your knees a few inches, and bracing your hands on the knees, keeping your arms straight. Proceed with the exercise as above. You may be tempted to close your eyes in order to concentrate more, but do not do so, as you may become dizzy.

"I got more pep, more energy. A lot more energy! There were times when I could hardly finish my lunch—I'd have to lie down and take a nap. I still take naps once in a while, but I don't need them like I used to. And I think it's the breathing exercises that's done that!"

—Josephine Vidmar (age 70)

CHAPTER 5

Chair Exercises

"Before I started Yoga, I'd wake up two or three times a night because my arms and legs would get stiff and I couldn't move. Now I sleep like a log and I don't get the cramps in my legs now as I did before."

—Ada Duffy (age 77)

In this chapter you will find some simple movements that you can do in a chair. Try a few first thing in the morning to get your blood moving and to relieve some of the stiffness built up during the night. Use a sturdy chair with a straight back. When you sit in the chair with your hips against the chair back, your feet should rest flat on the floor. If your feet don't touch and you can't find a shorter chair, place a sturdy support such as a telephone book under your feet.

Many of these exercises can also be done sitting on the edge of your bed or on the step of a swimming pool. If you sit on the edge of your bed, your feet must be able to rest firmly on the floor, and if you're in the pool, your feet must be flat on the bottom or on another step of the pool.

The first several exercises (pp. 65–71) are warm-ups that will improve circulation, gently begin to stretch your joints, and exercise the large muscles in your body. These can also be done standing.

Read over the instructions completely before you try an exercise, and keep your book near you. Always follow the instructions step by step; it is especially important to breathe in and out exactly as instructed so you get the most benefit from the simple movements. Most exercises call for you to repeat the movement three times. If that's too much at first, repeat only once or twice. Never strain; if it hurts, you've gone too far. If you keep your book nearby as you exercise, you will be able to check the instructions frequently; the spiral binding allows you to lay the book flat for easy reference.

Many exercises begin with the instruction to "Breathe in and out three times." Remember always to breathe through your nose, and fill your lungs deeply and slowly. When you take time for this breath pattern, you will increase the amount of oxygen you take in as you exercise, resulting in a brighter mind and a more attentive performance of the exercise.

Sometimes you will find one or the other nostril blocked. You can unclog this blockage in order to breathe freely through both nostrils using the technique described on p. 56.

Most exercises have a holding point at which you are instructed to "Hold for a count of three." Depending upon your stamina, hold for a quick count or a longer count. The idea is to make it a habit to include some period of holding each position, no matter how briefly. This will intensify the effects of the exercise.

Rest frequently during your exercise routine even if you don't feel tired. Frequent rests force you to pace yourself, give your body a chance to recover from any strenuous movements, and make sure that you don't injure yourself. Resting also allows you to develop a greater appreciation and respect for your body.

Frequently ask yourself how a particular movement makes you feel. This will encourage you to pay more attention to your body and will help you avoid strain by becoming more aware of how your body feels at all times. You might wish to keep a diary of the changes you have noticed as a result of your practice.

Do these exercises any time of day for a quick energy boost for body and mind. Many people have discovered that they can easily do some Easy Does It Yoga exercises and breathing techniques while they are watching television. This is a great way to keep fit without missing your favorite programs, and it keeps you from becoming sleepy or stiff. Similarly, if you work at a desk all day, doing a few exercises every hour or so will improve your concentration and alertness while improving circulation and preventing stiff joints—and will be much more beneficial than a coffee break.

> "Whenever I'm just sitting I try to do some Yoga—I never waste time just sitting watching TV. Instead of just sitting there all slouched over, I do leg lifts, knee squeezes, and the bending-over ones. I do my foot flaps and breathing and twisting. It limbers you up while you watch TV. And you know, after exercising, you feel better instead of all tired. You feel like getting up and doing something or going out."
> —Jeanne Hrovat (age 66)

Remember to read through the entire exercise before you try it. The exercises are organized from the simplest ones to those requiring more strength and stamina. Refer back to chapter 3 for suggested routines to start with. You can always add or subtract exercises either to give yourself more of a challenge or to make your routine easier.

ARM REACH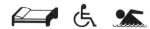

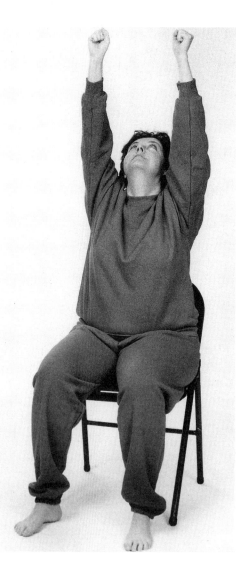

How Will This Exercise Help?

Strengthens arm muscles for carrying and lifting. Helps limber shoulders so you can reach higher over your head. Improves breathing and heart function. Tightens arm muscles.

Special Notes

If you have exceptionally stiff or sore shoulders, such as with severe arthritis, lift only as high as you can comfortably. If you have severe hypertension or a pacemaker, be very cautious and start with the variation, lifting one arm at a time.

1. Sit up straight, with your arms loose at your sides. Breathe in and out three times through your nose.
2. Slowly breathe in as you raise both arms in a wide circle to the sides and up toward the ceiling. (Note: This movement should be coordinated with one complete inhalation. If you find that you have completely filled your lungs before your arms reach the top position, try breathing a little more slowly.) Remember to breathe through your nose. Look up.
3. Make fists and hold your breath as you push your fists up toward the ceiling. Keep arms straight. Hold for a count of three.
4. Breathe out as you lower your arms. Relax. How did that feel?
5. Repeat twice more.

Variation

Lift one arm at a time, using the same breathing pattern: Breathe in as you lift the arm; hold as you push the fist up and count to three. Relax. Start with one on each side; work up to three on each side.

"I do the Arm Reaches every day. It helps my bursitis."
　　　　　　　　　　　　　　　　—Mae Norris (age 84)

"Every morning I'd have terrible indigestion. And you know what's helped? I do those Arm Reaches with my fists up toward the ceiling and that gets rid of it right away!"
—Katrina Price (age 68)

ELBOW ROLL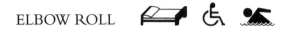

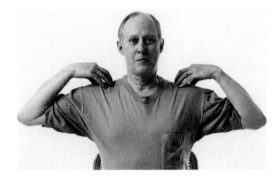

How Will This Exercise Help?

Strengthens shoulder and upper arm muscles so you can raise your arms higher. Improves your range of motion so that you can do your daily activities more easily. Improves respiration and heart function.

Special Notes

Your elbows should move in large, smooth circles. Move slowly. If your hands can't reach the top of your shoulders, place them on your chest as high as possible without strain. If you have severe joint problems or hypertension, rest and lower your arms after each rotation.

1. Sit up straight in your chair with feet flat on the floor. Breathe in and out three times, then breathe normally throughout this exercise.
2. Touch the top of your shoulders with your fingertips, and raise your elbows straight out to your sides.
3. Slowly circle your elbows forward three times, slowly, then rest. Now lift your elbows out again and circle them backward, three times, slowly.
3. Repeat if desired.

Variations

• Rotate the elbows in small circles with fingertips on the chest.
• Elbow Touch: With fingers on shoulders, bring elbows together in front of the body, breathing out, and stretch them back horizontally as if they could touch in the back, breathing in. Repeat three times.

"I had a pain in my shoulder. It was like an ice pick. This is the exercise that really helped."

—Gene Roy (age 62)

SHOULDER ROLL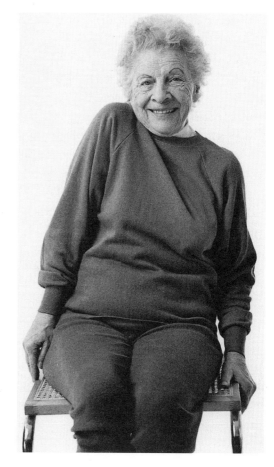

How Will This Exercise Help?

Strengthens and limbers muscles of the shoulders, upper torso, and arms that are used for reaching and while driving. Improves range of motion in the shoulders, which helps relieve muscle tension in your upper back.

Special Notes

Make every movement slow and controlled, while trying to rotate your shoulders as fully as possible. Avoid painful, extreme movements.

You can rest your hands in your lap or let your arms hang loosely at your sides. As you rotate your shoulders, keep your neck and head steady and relaxed. If your shoulders are quite stiff or painful, massage them gently before doing this exercise (see p. 73).

1. Sit up straight in your chair and let your arms and shoulders relax. Breathe in and out three times, then breathe normally throughout the exercise.
2. Lift your right shoulder (keeping your arm and hand relaxed) and roll it forward, down, gently back, and up in a circular motion. Continue circling your shoulder twice more forward, then relax and shake out your arm.
3. Now raise your left shoulder and rotate it forward three times. Relax and shake out.
4. Rotate right shoulder three times backward, then relax and shake out your arm.
5. Rotate left shoulder three times backward, then relax and shake out.

Variation: Double Shoulder Roll

1. Letting your arms hang loosely at your sides or rest in your lap, lift both shoulders and roll them forward

three times. Rest, then roll both shoulders backward three times.
2. When this exercise becomes easy for you, do it while tightening all your arm muscles and making fists.

"Last week I actually reached up and painted my awnings and house myself. I hadn't been able to do something like that for a long time. But since I started my Yoga, I just reached right up there and didn't even get sore from all that stretching and craning my neck. I did it all myself!"
—Dora Richardson (age 70)

THROAT TIGHTENER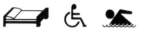

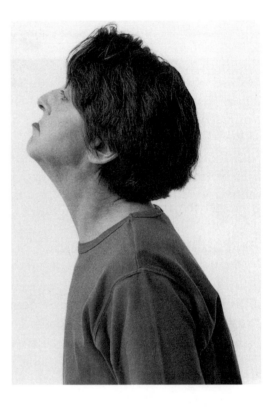

How Will This Exercise Help?

Increases circulation to the head. Improves self-confidence and mood. Stretches and tones the muscles in the neck and throat. Keeps neck looking youthful by helping to prevent double chin and wrinkles.

Special Notes

If you have a disk problem in your neck, do this exercise very gently; be careful not to strain.

1. Sit up straight and place your hands on your hips.
2. Take a deep breath in, through your nose. Hold your breath and thrust your chin gently forward, stretching the muscles of your throat. Your head will be slightly tipped back.
3. Breathe out and relax back.
4. Repeat, thrusting your chin to the right, relaxing, then to the left. Do a total of three chin thrusts in each of the three directions.

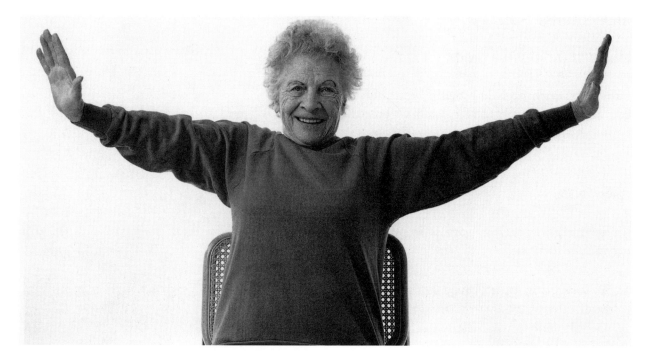

ARM CIRCLES

How Will This Exercise Help?

Limbers the shoulder joints and strengthens shoulder and upper back muscles, making it easier to perform everyday activities such as reaching overhead and carrying groceries, children, or other loads. Strengthens and tightens the muscles and skin of the upper arms. Improves respiration and heart function.

Special Notes

If you have arthritis or bursitis in your shoulder joints, use caution; start with smaller movements.

1. Sit up straight in your chair with feet flat on the floor and arms at your sides. Breathe in and out three times, then breathe normally throughout this exercise.
2. Stretch your arms out to the sides at shoulder height. Push your palms outward, fingers together, as if stopping traffic on either side of you.
3. Slowly rotate your arms in a large circle forward, rotating your arm as far up and around as you can. Do 3–5 slow circles.
4. Relax and rest, then do 3–5 circles rotating in the opposite direction.

ARM SWING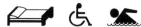

How Will This Exercise Help?

Expands the rib cage, improving breathing. Invigorates and energizes the body. Helps relieve breathing problems and depression. Improves heart function.

Special Notes

If you have arthritis or bursitis in your shoulder, be careful not to strain.

1. Sit forward in your chair. Breathe in and out three times. Stretch your arms straight ahead, level with your shoulders, and breathe out (A). Your back will feel slightly slouched forward.
2. Start to breathe in deeply and push your chest and stomach forward as you open your arms wide to the sides and back as far as you can behind you without straining (B). Your back will be very slightly arched.
3. Breathe out as you bring your arms together in front of you, slouching forward again. Rest and relax.
4. Repeat 3–5 times.

Variations

If your arms are quite weak, start with one repetition only, then rest. You can also do this exercise in bed, lying on your side, working with one arm at a time; work up to three repetitions on each side.

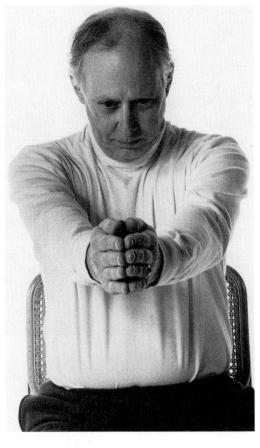

A

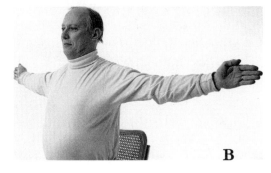

B

NECK STRETCHES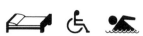

How Will This Exercise Help?

Helps to loosen up the joints and muscles in your neck so you can look behind you when necessary while driving and at other times. Gently stretches and strengthens the muscles at the sides and back of the neck to avoid headaches and neck pain due to stiff, tight muscles.

Special Notes

Your neck is very vulnerable to extreme, jerky, and forced movements. Always move slowly and gently in this exercise, bending the neck only until the muscles feel stretched; never bend your neck to the point of pain. Never let your head drop backward. If you feel any dizziness, racing pulse, or pain, stop immediately and rest. If you have disk problems in your neck, do only the variation in which the head is gently turned from side to side.

It's important to keep your shoulders relaxed at all times so you are only moving your head; many students tend to lift their shoulders toward their ears. Constantly remind yourself to relax your shoulders. Note that your hands are to be held on your neck at all times; this forms a supportive "collar" that will help prevent injury to your neck.

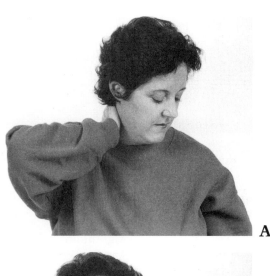

A

1. Sit up straight in your chair. Breathe normally throughout this exercise.
2. Gently bend your head down and to the left without bending your upper back, so your chin comes down toward your collarbone while looking to the left as far as you can. Put your right hand up to the right side of your neck to feel the muscles stretching (A). Hold for a few seconds, breathing normally.
3. Bring your head back up straight and bend it down and toward the right. Push your chin down toward your collarbone while looking to the right as far as you can. Put your left hand on the left side of your neck and feel the muscles stretching tight.
4. Relax. Massage your neck with both hands (see p. 73).

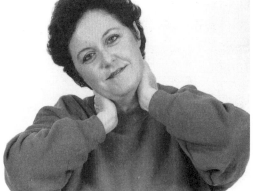

B

5. Next, place both hands on your neck and gently tilt your head to the right (B), bring it back up straight and tilt down toward the left. Repeat twice more.
6. Still keeping your hands on your neck, look straight ahead and slowly turn your head to look over your left shoulder (C). Slowly turn back and all the way over to the right shoulder.
7. Repeat twice more.

Variations

- If these movements feel fine, try a gentle rotation: Slowly lower your right ear toward your right shoul-

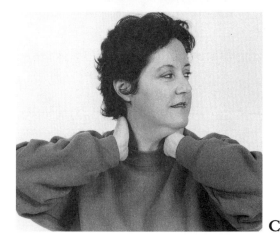

C

der, next lower your chin toward your chest, then gently bring your left ear toward your left shoulder, and slowly bring your head up straight. Relax, then repeat the rotation in the opposite direction. Repeat 1–3 times to each side.

- If you have disk problems or pain in your neck, do only very slight movements of the turning variation (Step 6) and be sure that your neck is supported at all times with both hands.

"I have arthritis in my back and neck so I could never turn when I was in the car. I always had to use the mirror to back up. Since I've done my Yoga, I can go all the way back, with my neck, like this!"

—Jeanne Hrovat (age 66)

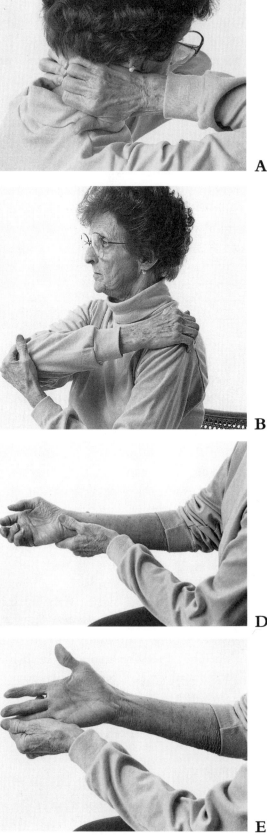

A

B

MASSAGE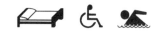

How Will This Exercise Help?

Helps remove stiffness in the joints and muscles and improves circulation, making exercise easier and more pleasant, and reducing strain and injury. Helps put you in touch with your physical body, improving self-esteem.

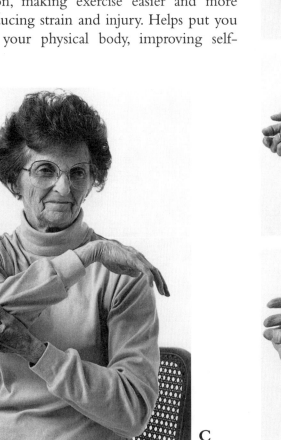

C

D

E

Special Notes

The point of this exercise is not to press hard with the hands and fingers but simply to increase warmth in the joints, which will help loosen them. Use your whole hand when rubbing a joint, not just the fingers. Massage each joint for at least 15 seconds. It's a good idea to get into the habit of massaging your joints several times during your exercise session as well as at other times during the day. It is easy and enjoyable to massage your joints while watching television or resting in bed, for instance.

To massage your neck: Rub the right side and back of your neck with your right hand (A). Use your palm and rub gently for at least 15 seconds. Repeat on the left side, using your left palm.

To massage your shoulders: Start by supporting your right elbow in your left hand. With your right hand, gently rub your left shoulder, using your whole hand—not just the fingers (B). Rub the entire joint. Don't press hard with your fingers; the point is to warm up the joint with your palm, not to dig in.

To massage your elbow: Using your palm, rub all around your elbow joint (C).

To massage your hands and fingers: With your left thumb, rub your right palm and wrist, using a circular motion (D). Then, starting at the base of your right thumb, use your left thumb on top and left fingers underneath to rub firmly in a circular motion all over and around the joint. Move up the thumb rubbing the same way at each knuckle joint. Repeat with each of your fingers, starting from the base of each (E).

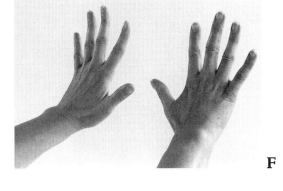

F

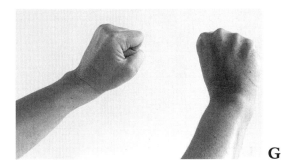

G

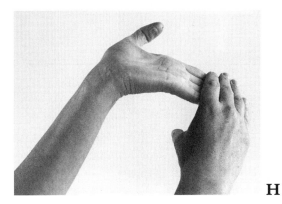

H

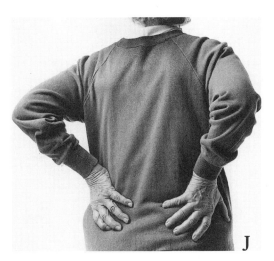

J

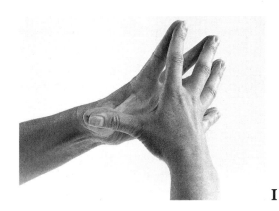

I

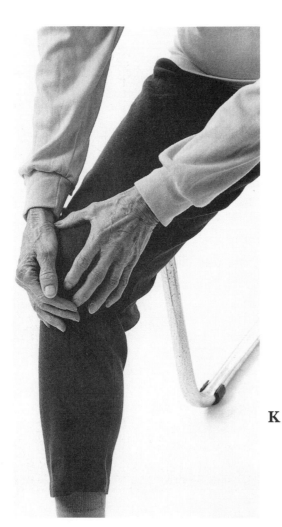

K

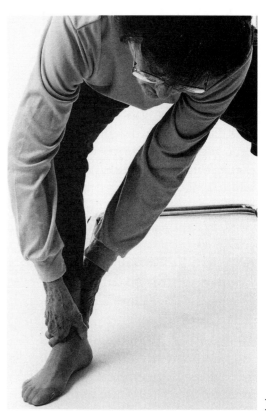

L

Loosen your finger and wrist joints further: Spread your fingers wide apart (F), then make fists (G). Repeat several times. Press the fingers of one hand back using the opposite hand (H). Repeat on the opposite side. Make a "steeple" with your fingers (I) and press the fingers together.

To massage your lower back: Place both hands on your lower back and rub firmly up and down all the way to the tailbone, using your whole hand (J).

To massage your knees and ankles: Massage one knee at a time. Place both hands on your knee. Rub up with one hand and down with the other hand simultaneously in a semicircular motion over the entire knee area (K). Massage ankles similarly (L).

"My wife likes to massage her hands while we watch TV. It really has helped her. She took the book and showed it to her doctors, and they both really approved. The one said, 'Take this home and use it!' "

—Willard Weeks (age 79)

FACIAL EXERCISES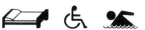

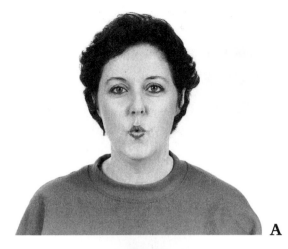

A

How Will This Exercise Help?

Stretches and tightens facial muscles. Helps lower inhibitions and strengthen vocal cords. Also helps to prevent "monkey lines" around the mouth and nose and make eyes bright by forcing oxygen into the facial muscles. Helps keep lips full and attractive.

Special Notes

Have fun! In the vowel exercise, exaggerate the sounds in order to stretch your facial muscles, and make the vowels as loud as possible.

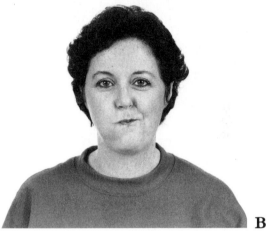

B

Vowel Exercise

1. Sit up straight in your chair. Put your hands on your hips.
2. Say "AAAAA" (as in the word "say") . . . "EEEEE" . . . "IIIII" (as in "eye") . . . "OOOOO" . . . "UUUUU" ("yooo") (A). Exaggerate the movement of your lips, jaws, and throat to make the sounds full, round, and rich (A).
3. Repeat 3–5 times.

Cheek Fill Exercise

1. Sit up straight in your chair. Put your hands on your hips.
2. Fill your cheeks with air, and move the air from side to side and up and down several times, holding your breath in (B).
3. Breathe out and rest for a moment.
4. Fill your cheeks with air again, hold your breath, and this time move the air around in a circle, two or three times in each direction.

THE LION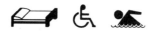

How Will This Exercise Help?

Invigorates and energizes, while providing emotional release and lowering self-consciousness. Improves the complexion, facial expression, and voice by releasing tension in facial muscles. Helps break the cycle of depression.

Special Notes

Ham it up, and exaggerate the movements in this exercise. Have fun! To do the exercise in bed, lie on your back with knees bent and feet flat several inches apart. Place hands on thighs and proceed with Step 2.

1. Sit up straight with your feet flat on the floor.
2. Spread your fingers apart like a lion's paws and grip your knees.
3. Lean forward slightly and take a deep breath through your nose.
4. Open your eyes wide, raise your eyebrows, stick out your tongue, and roar fiercely like a lion!
5. Repeat three times.

FROG POSE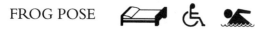

How Will This Exercise Help?

Improves flexibility and circulation in the spine. Improves respiration and also promotes normal bowel function.

Special Notes

Be sure to move slowly and carefully. Be especially careful to bend your neck very slowly and gently.

1. Sit up straight, with your knees slightly separated and your feet flat on the floor. Breathe in and out three times.
2. Grasp your knees with your hands.

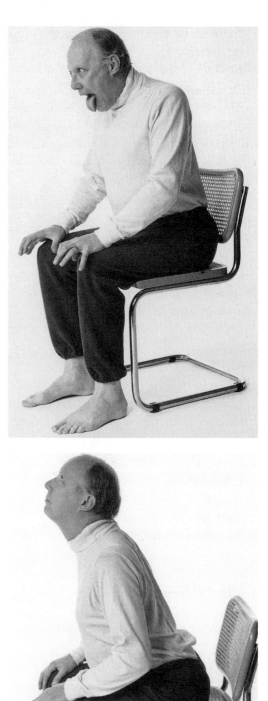

A

3. Breathe in deeply as you arch your back and look up, leaning forward slightly (A).
4. Hold your breath for a count of three.
5. Breathe out as you bend the opposite way, rounding your back and tucking your chin into your chest (B). Hold your breath for a count of three. Breathe in and relax.
6. Repeat twice more.

SIDE STRETCH

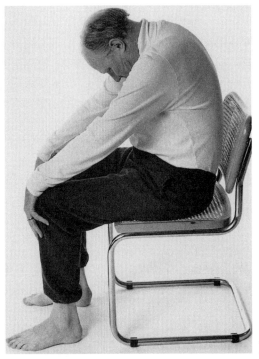

B

How Will This Exercise Help?

Strengthens muscles and increases limberness of the spine and hip joints. Good for toning of the waistline. Helps breathing problems by stretching and strengthening respiratory muscles. Improves balance.

Special Notes

If you have weak back and side muscles, instead of reaching over your head, hold on to the chair with one hand while you bend to the opposite side. Bend only as far as you can comfortably at first until you are more confident.

1. Sit up straight. Let your arms relax at your sides. Breathe in and out three times.
2. Take a deep breath in and bend toward your right side, stretching your right arm down toward the floor and bending your left arm up and over your head.
3. Hold your breath for a count of three.
4. Breathe out and return to your starting position. Relax.
5. Take a deep breath in and bend toward your left side, stretching your left arm down toward the floor and bending your right arm up and over your head.
6. Hold your breath for a count of three.
7. Breathe out and return to your starting position. Relax.
8. Repeat twice more on each side, alternating.

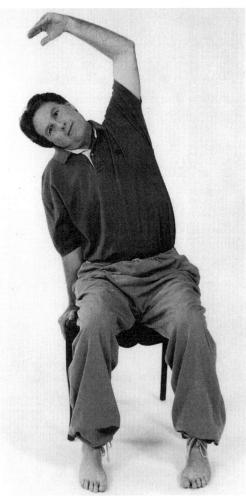

Variation

This exercise can be done standing, holding on to a sturdy support. It is especially effective done in the pool. Hold on to the edge or a railing with one hand and reach up and over with the other hand, breathing as instructed above.

ELBOW TWIST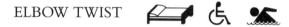

How Will This Exercise Help?

Improves circulation to spine and brain. Limbers vertebrae in the spine to help you look behind you when you back out of a driveway, or at other times. Strengthens neck, shoulder, and arm muscles. Improves breathing. This is a good warm-up exercise for the Seated Twist, which follows.

Special Notes

Be sure not to strain, and twist only a short distance at first. Never force your body to twist farther than it can comfortably.

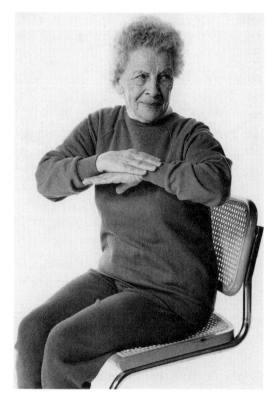

1. Sit up straight in your chair with feet flat on the floor. Breathe in and out three times through your nose.
2. Lift your arms, bend your elbows, and place one hand flat on top of the other hand at chest height about six inches away from your body.
3. Breathe in, looking forward. Breathe out as you twist gently toward the left, leading with your left elbow. Hold your breath out for a count of three.
4. Breathe in and turn back to the front.
5. Breathe out as you twist gently to the right, leading with your right elbow. Hold your breath out for a count of three. Breathe in and turn back to the front. Rest.
6. Repeat twice more to each side, alternating sides.

SEATED TWIST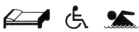

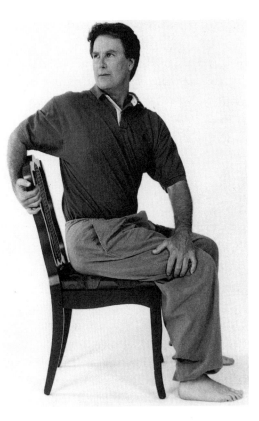

How Will This Exercise Help?

Improves circulation to spine and brain. Limbers the vertebrae in the spine so you can look behind you when backing up your car, or at other times. Strengthens neck, shoulder, and upper arm muscles. Improves eyesight. Strengthens lungs.

Special Notes

Many people are quite stiff when they attempt this motion for the first time. Be sure not to strain, and twist only a short distance at first. Never force your body to twist farther than it can comfortably.

1. Sit up straight in your chair with feet flat on the floor. Breathe in and out three times.
2. Place your right hand on the outside of your left knee. Place your left arm across the back of the chair, or inside the back of the chair, or in any comfortable position that pulls the left arm back slightly. Grasp the chair back or seat firmly.
3. Sit up straight, and breathe in completely.
4. Breathe out as you slowly turn your torso toward the left as far as you can. Pull slightly with your right hand to get the greatest stretch. Turn your head as far toward the left as you can, and look to the left with your eyes.
5. Hold the position and your breath out for a count of three.
6. Breathe in as you slowly return to face front. Relax.
7. Switch arms and repeat the exercise to the right. (Note: This exercise is done only once in each direction.)

Variations

If you have severe arthritis in your shoulders and find it painful to twist your shoulders, simply place both hands on the opposite leg instead of twisting one arm behind your chair. This will still strengthen your arms and shoulders and provide a gentle twist until you can manage the complete exercise.

> *"My wife and I do a lot of Yoga exercises together in our chairs while we watch TV. We especially like the twisting ones. I had arthritis and cramps down in my ankles and the tops of my feet. I can't explain how it helps, but it helps all the way into my toes and everything."*
> —Willard Weeks (age 79)

SEATED LEG LIFT AND FOOT FLAPS

How Will This Exercise Help?

Limbers the hip joint, strengthens the abdominal, hip, and knee muscles, and stretches the muscles in the back of the legs. This exercise will improve your walking and stair-climbing ability by strengthening your legs and improving your balance and confidence. If your balance is uncertain, this exercise can help you avoid falls.

Special Notes

If you have arthritis in your hips, do only one repetition on each side at first and try to repeat the exercise several times during the day. Breathe deeply at all times during the exercise as instructed.

Sit with your hips and back pressed against the chair back to start, as this will provide support for weak back muscles (though the leg will not lift as high in this position; in the completed pose, the thigh should be lifted off the chair seat). After a while, you can try sitting forward slightly, maintaining a straight back during the exercise but not leaning against the chair back. Naturally, if you have disk or severe muscular problems in your back, support yourself against the chair back throughout. This exercise can be done in bed by lying down flat and lifting the legs as described. Sometimes leg cramps are a sign of protein deficiency (see Diet and Nutrition chapter for more details).

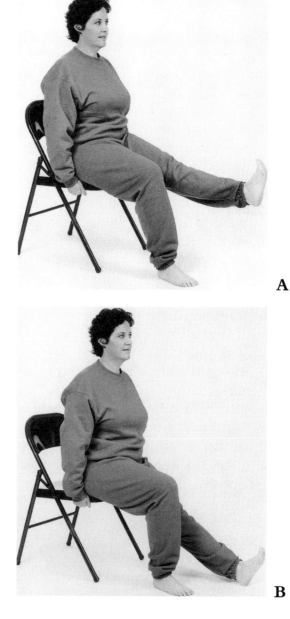

A

B

SEATED LEG LIFTS

1. Sit up straight with hips against the back of your chair, and hold tightly to the side of your chair seat. Breathe in and out three times.
2. Breathe out all your air.
3. Breathe in and hold your breath in as you straighten your right knee and lift your leg to waist level—or as high as you can without straining (A). Hold for a count of three.
4. Breathe out as you slowly lower your leg to the floor and relax.
5. Repeat with the left leg, and then do two more repetitions on each leg, alternating legs.

Variations

When the exercise above is no longer a challenge for you, try to lift your extended leg up above the level of the chair seat and hold for a count of three.

If the Seated Leg Lift is too difficult for you at first, begin by doing the Foot Flap and Ankle Rotation every day. These warm-ups limber and strengthen ankle and calf muscles, and improve circulation in the extremities.

> *"My knees used to be so arthritic. I used to have to hold on to the banister and just go downstairs like a little baby. I had to put both feet on the step, hold on, and then slowly go to the next stair. I felt so dopey. Now I can go up and down the stairs almost normally. It still hurts a little bit, but I can go down without holding on."*
> —Jeanne Hrovat (age 66)

FOOT FLAP AND ANKLE ROTATION

1. Sit up straight with your hips against the seat back. Hold on to the chair bottom with both hands. Breathe normally throughout this exercise.
2. Stretch your left leg forward and rest the heel on the floor.
3. Gently push your toes forward and pull them back (B), several times, stretching as far as possible in each direction.
4. Rotate your ankle, three times in one direction, then three times in the other direction.
5. Rest a moment, then stretch your right foot forward and repeat: Push your toes forward and back several times, then rotate in each direction a few times.

"It was very hard for me to get in and out of cars, even big ones. I always had to be helped—no, pulled out! But since my Yoga, that problem's gone because I can move now!
—Helen Gould (age 65)

SEATED KNEE SQUEEZE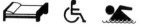

How Will This Exercise Help?

Limbers the neck, hip, knee, and ankle joints; strengthens the elbow and hip joints; and improves oxygenation of the blood. Stretches the muscles and joints used in walking and stair climbing, as well as muscles in the arms and shoulders used to lift and carry things. This exercise also stimulates digestion and can help relieve constipation and gas.

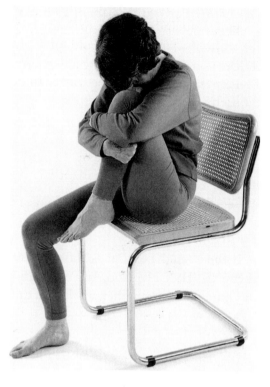

Special Notes

This exercise is somewhat strenuous, so if you have severe high blood pressure, check with your doctor before trying it. Never hold the compression for more than 3 seconds.

If you have arthritic or painful knee joints, do this exercise by grasping your thigh close to your knee with both hands, instead of squeezing the knee.

See p. 116 for a variation of this exercise that can be done in bed.

1. Sit up straight, away from the back of your chair, with your arms at your sides. Do not lean against the back of your chair. Breathe in and out three times through your nose.
2. Slowly breathe out as much air as possible.
3. Now breathe in, lift your right knee up high, and squeeze it to your chest with both arms. (If you can't reach around with both arms, grasp the knee with both hands instead.)
4. Hold for a count of three.
5. As you slowly breathe out, relax your arms and lower your leg to the floor.
6. Repeat with the left leg. Rest. Then repeat twice more with each leg, alternating sides.

Variations

After you have mastered the basic technique, point your toes down toward the floor as you lift and squeeze.

After further practice, during the squeeze, lower your forehead toward your raised knee.

"I had to take something all the time for constipation. Drawing up the knees and squeezing has been good for me. I haven't had to take anything in seven months. Sure has saved my husband and me some drugstore money. Not only that, but I love cheese, and now I can eat cheese again!"
— Annie Mae Johnson (age 63)

"I had a gas pocket here on my left side giving me terrible pain which lasted for three days. I even went to the emergency room at the hospital one night, it was so bad, but they didn't help me get relief. I was in such misery with the pain. Then I remembered and did some of my Yoga exercises— Elbow Rolls, Folded Pose, and that Knee Squeeze. I started feeling so much better right then! I just couldn't believe it. Now I hardly ever get that gas, and I used to have it all the time. If it acts like it's coming back, I just get in my bed and do those Knee Squeezes."
— Emma Mae Mays (age 63)

LAUGHING BICYCLE

How Will This Exercise Help?

Invigorates and oxygenates the body and brain and relaxes all the muscle groups. Eliminates apathy, depression, and irritability—it's a wonderful relief from the "blues." Reduces feelings of stress and anxiety. Increases alertness and interest in life. Improves heart function.

Special Notes

This exercise is guaranteed to lift even the bleakest mood.

1. Make loose fists and move arms freely in circles as if you are pedaling a bicycle with your hands.
2. Move legs too, leaning back in your chair (A).

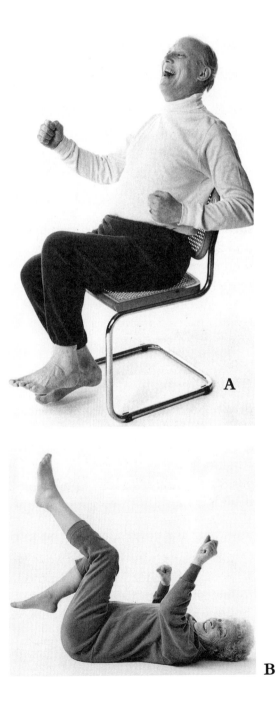

A

B

3. Laugh out loud for about 30 seconds. Make the sound of laughing, and soon you'll really be laughing!

Variations

You can also do this exercise lying on your back in bed or on the floor (B).

"When I started Yoga I couldn't bend my leg and knee—had arthritis and rheumatism in it for about eighteen years. Yoga sure helped. It's really better."

—Ada Duffy (age 77)

FOLDED POSE AND VARIATION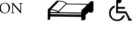

How Will This Exercise Help?

Increases limberness in the vertebrae of the neck and back; gently stretches the muscles of the neck, back, and hips; increases blood supply to the head, bringing fresh oxygen to your brain. This exercise will help gradually reduce back pain caused by tension or muscle weakness. It also helps to improve breathing and strengthens the heart.

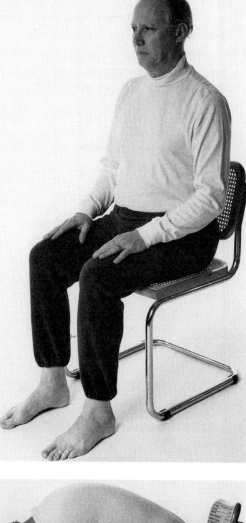

A

Special Notes

If you are afraid of falling forward, do the Folded Pose Variation (below) until you gain confidence. If you experience dizziness or heavy pounding in your temples, don't bend as far forward.

1. Sit up straight, with your lower back pressed against the back of your chair and your feet firmly on the floor. If your feet don't touch the floor, place a pillow under your feet as shown in photo (D).
2. Put your knees together, and put your hands on your knees (A).
3. Slowly take in a deep breath through your nose.

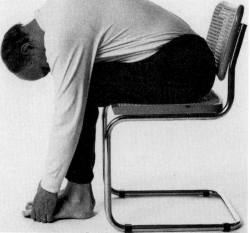

B

4. As you slowly breathe out, curl your head and spine toward your knees, bending forward to touch your chest to your thighs.

5. If this feels comfortable, let your arms drop to the sides of your legs, hands loosely reaching toward the floor. Be sure to let your head and neck relax completely (B).

6. Hold for a count of three.

7. Breathe in and come up slowly, supporting yourself by putting your hands back on your knees. Breathe out. Rest and relax. (Note: This exercise is done only once.)

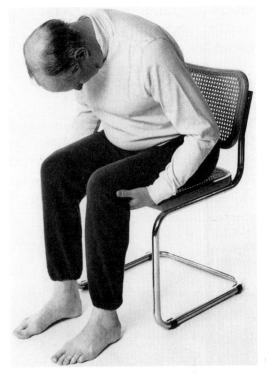

C

Variations

If you have high blood pressure and your doctor has told you not to lower your head below your heart, substitute the following exercise:

FOLDED POSE VARIATION

1. Sit up straight. Do not lean against the back of your chair. Breathe in and out three times.

2. Place hands under your thighs near your knees, and put your knees together.

3. Slowly take in a deep breath and hold it for a count of three.

4. Breathe out as you drop your chin toward your chest and continue curling your spine forward as far as you can (C). This entire movement should take only about 5 seconds.

5. Hold your breath out for a count of three.

6. Now breathe in and straighten, uncurling your spine from the bottom up.

7. Repeat twice more.

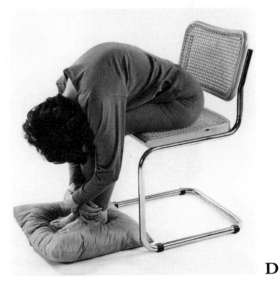

D

SEATED FULL BEND BREATH
AND SUPPORTED FULL BEND
BREATH

How Will This Exercise Help?

Stretches major muscle groups in legs and back, stimulates the breathing and circulatory systems, and improves coordination. Increases overall fitness, helps improve posture, and facilitates bending and reaching movements. May also help to tighten waistline. Keeps you tall.

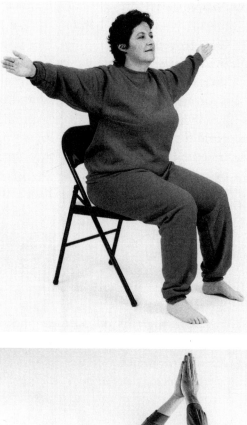

A

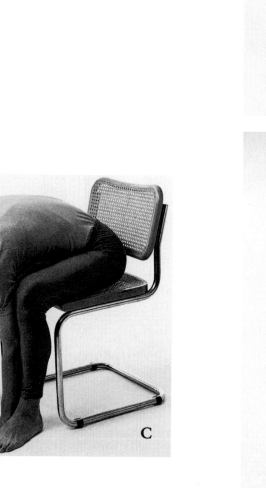

C

B

Special Notes

Breathe smoothly and slowly throughout this exercise; always breathe through your nose.

Make sure your legs and feet are firmly in place and that your hips are pressed against the seat back to avoid any danger of falling forward. If you feel unsteady, start with the Supported Full Bend Breath (below) until you are more confident about bending forward.

1. Sit up straight in your chair with knees apart and feet firmly placed on the floor. Rest your lower back against the chair back for support. Breathe in and out three times.
2. Breathe out completely, then breathe in as you raise your arms to the sides in a wide circle (A) and overhead.
3. Look up and hold for a quick count of three (B).
4. Breathe out as you tuck your head and bend forward slowly, reaching your arms forward toward the floor. Breathe out all the way forward (C).
5. Hold your breath out for a count of three.
6. Slowly breathe in as you raise your arms to the sides and overhead again as in Step 2. Look up and hold for a count of three.
7. Breathe out and relax your arms. Rest.
8. Repeat twice more.

SUPPORTED FULL BEND BREATH

1. Sit straight in your chair with your knees apart, feet firmly placed on the floor, and hips pressed against the chair back. Breathe in and out three times.
2. Hold on to your left knee with your left hand. Let your right arm hang down at your side.
3. Breathe out completely. Breathe in as you raise your right arm in a circle to the side and up over your head. Make a fist and look up (D). Hold your breath for a count of three.
4. As you start to breathe out, tuck your chin and slowly bend forward, reaching forward and down toward the floor with your right hand (E). Rest your chest on your thighs if possible; otherwise, relax your upper body as much as possible. Hold your breath out for a count of three.

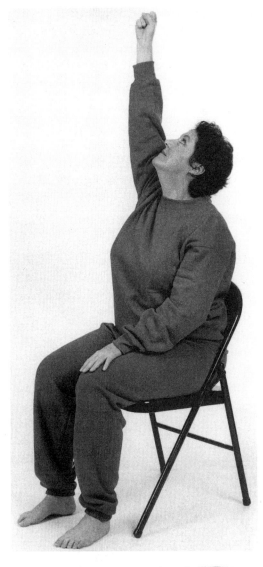

D

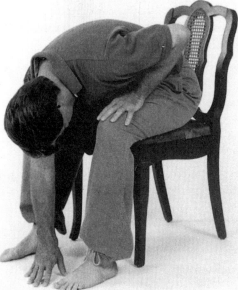

E

Chair Exercises • 87

5. Breathe in and come up, reaching forward and up toward the ceiling with your right arm. Slowly breathe out as you lower your arm down to your side. Rest.

6. Repeat on the opposite side, then repeat twice more on each side, alternating.

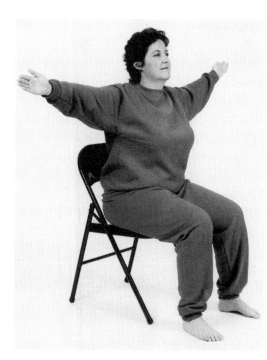

FULL BEND TWIST AND SUPPORTED FULL BEND TWIST

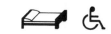

How Will This Exercise Help?

Stretches and strengthens muscles of the shoulders, arms, torso, and hip joints. Improves breathing. Makes it easier to bend, twist, and reach. Improves heart function.

A

Special Notes

This is a strenuous exercise, so be sure to move slowly and deliberately, aware of your body at all times. Breathe fully and deeply. Be sure legs and feet are firmly placed and hips are pressed against the seat back. If you have disk problems in your spine or neck, check with your doctor before trying this exercise.

1. Sit up straight with your arms at your sides and your knees and feet spread apart. Breathe in and out three times.

2. Breathe out as much as you can, then breathe in deeply as you raise both arms out to the sides and up to shoulder height (A).

3. Slowly breathe out as you bend forward to touch your *right* hand to your *left* foot (B). Your left arm points up toward the ceiling.

4. Breathe in and come back up straight with arms out to the sides.

5. Breathe out and relax your arms.

6. Repeat on the other side: Slowly breathe out as you bend forward to touch your *left* hand to your *right* foot. Your right arm points up toward the ceiling.

7. Breathe in and come back up straight with arms out to the sides.

8. Breathe out and relax your arms. Rest.

9. Repeat twice more on each side, alternating sides.

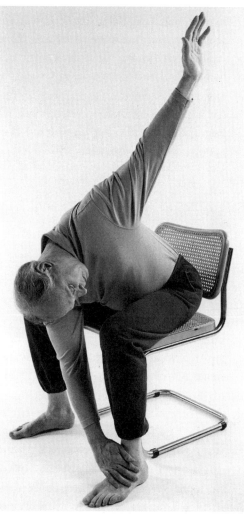

B

Variations

After mastering the movements of this exercise, turn your head and look at your upraised hand when you are in Step 3.

If you are afraid of falling or extremely weak, start with the Supported Full Bend Twist, below. For even more safety, place your chair facing your bed or a sturdy, soft chair; if you become dizzy while bending over, this extra support will keep you from falling.

SUPPORTED FULL BEND TWIST

1. Sit up straight with lower back against the chair back, knees apart and feet firmly placed. Place your left hand on your left knee. Breathe in and out three times.
2. Breathe in as you raise your right arm up and out to the side, shoulder height.
3. Slowly breathe out as you reach down toward your left foot with your right hand (C). Use your left hand on your knee for support.
4. Slowly breathe in as you come back up. Relax.
5. Repeat on the opposite side: Slowly breathe out as you reach down toward your right foot with your left hand. Use your right hand on your knee for support.
6. Slowly breathe in as you come back up. Relax.
7. Repeat twice more on each side, alternating.

ELBOW TO KNEE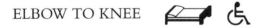

How Will This Exercise Help?

Stretches and strengthens back muscles and increases flexibility of the spine. Expands chest muscles, which helps to relieve breathing problems. Improves posture by strengthening back muscles.

Special Notes

If you have weak back muscles or lower back problems, take extra care not to strain with this twisting exercise.

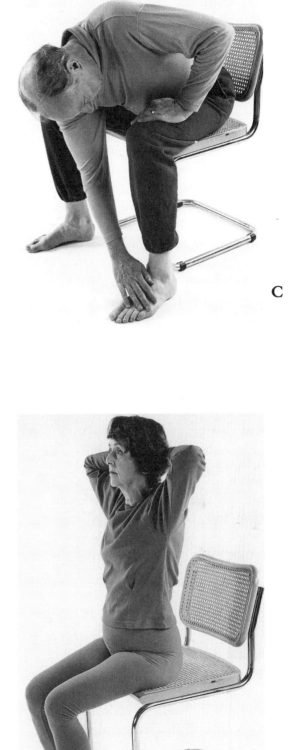

C

A

1. Sit up straight in your chair with your feet flat on the floor about a foot apart. Breathe in and out three times.
2. Clasp your hands behind your neck and breathe in completely (A).
3. As you breathe out, bend forward and twist slightly so your right elbow moves toward your left knee (B).
4. Hold your breath out for a count of three.
5. Breathe in and come back up. Relax.
6. Repeat on the opposite side: Clasp your hands behind your neck and breathe in completely.
7. As you breathe out, bend forward and twist slightly so your left elbow moves toward your right knee.
8. Hold your breath out for a count of three.
9. Breathe in and come back up. Relax.
10. Repeat twice more on each side, alternating.

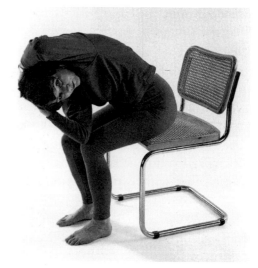

B

Variations

If you cannot clasp your hands behind your neck, you can do this exercise with fingers touching your shoulders instead.

SHOULDER TO KNEE

How Will This Exercise Help?

Limbers the spine and strengthens muscles in the back, side, and abdomen. Improves the functioning of the internal organs, particularly the heart, lungs, and kidneys.

Special Notes

This is a more strenuous version of the Elbow to Knee exercise. If you have neck or back problems, be especially careful with this exercise.

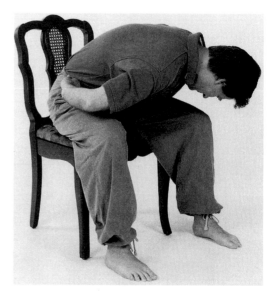

1. Sit up straight. Do not lean against the back of the chair. Place your feet flat on the floor. Rest your hands on your hips. Breathe in and out three times through your nose.
2. Breathe in completely.

3. Breathe out as you bend forward and lean toward the left, reaching with your right shoulder toward your left knee.
4. Hold your breath for a count of three.
5. Breathe in and come up. Relax.
6. Repeat on the opposite side: Breathe in completely. Breathe out as you bend forward and lean toward the right, reaching with your left shoulder toward your right knee.
7. Hold your breath for a count of three.
8. Breathe in and come up. Relax.
9. Repeat twice more on each side, alternating.

Variations

If you are afraid of falling, you can do this exercise holding onto the chair seat at first instead of placing hands on hips.

CHAPTER 6

Standing Exercises

"I used to have to rock back and forth five or six times to get out of this chair. I have new strength in my legs now and I can get right up."

—Emma Mae Mays (age 63)

In this chapter you will learn several exercises that you can do standing. Try them throughout the day to keep your circulation moving and your joints active. Standing exercises will also help strengthen the bones of your legs. Have a sturdy support nearby, such as the back of a sturdy chair, in case your balance becomes unsteady. Be sure you are standing on a nonskid surface. You will strengthen your feet, ankles, and calves more if you practice these exercises in bare feet; however, if you feel unbalanced without shoes, or have weak ankles, you may practice with shoes on at first.

Get in the habit of practicing the standing exercises at home at any time of day. For instance, while talking on the telephone, you can hold on to a sturdy support and practice the Strut, the Leg Lifts, or a Standing Reach.

Most exercises are done in groups of three repetitions. Always rest 30 seconds after you first try each exercise to be sure you are not straining.

All the standing exercises will strengthen your legs and back—essential for getting down on the floor and up again as well as walking and stair climbing. By practicing some of these exercises every day, you will build confidence and strength for all your daily activities.

If you have access to a heated pool, try a few of these exercises standing in the shallow end holding on to a railing or the edge of the pool. Be sure to breathe correctly and do the same number of repetitions on each side. Doing these exercises in water increases the resistance, which helps build muscle tone.

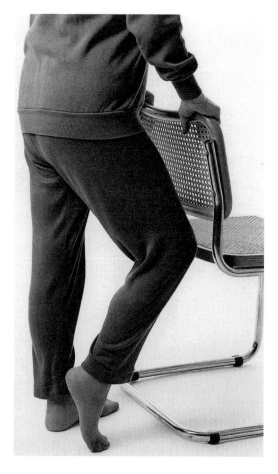

STRUT

How Will This Exercise Help?

Strengthens and relaxes leg muscles to help you in walking and climbing stairs. Helps you build the coordination and strength needed to get down on the floor and back up safely. Helps prevent and relieve leg cramps. Builds ankle and leg strength.

1. Stand behind a chair, holding on to the chair back with both hands. Your feet should be at a comfortable, stable distance apart. Breathe normally.
2. Keeping the balls and toes of both feet in contact with the floor at all times, bend one knee slightly and then the other, lifting your heels and shifting your weight slowly from one foot to the other. Relax your spine so that it flexes slightly from side to side and your hips sway. Your whole body moves gracefully as you strut as if swaying to a slow, dancing beat.

"If it hadn't been for Yoga, I might not be walking by now. I could hardly move my legs. Then I started Yoga, and that brought the stiffness out of my joints."

—Jim Chesser (age 77)

ANKLE STRENGTHENERS

How Will This Exercise Help?

Strengthens feet, ankles, and calves, and improves balance; this increases confidence in walking, stair climbing, and other activities. Helps to prevent and relieve leg cramps.

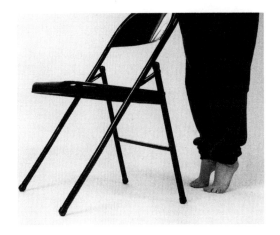

Special Notes

If your ankles are weak and you find it difficult to hold the position with heels raised, practice the exercise simply by pushing up on your toes and coming right back down again until you are stronger.

1. Stand behind a chair with your feet together. Hold on with both hands and look straight ahead. Breathe in and out three times through your nose.
2. Breathe in and lift your heels while coming up on your toes. Hold your breath and the position for a count of three.
3. Breathe out and come back down on flat feet. Rest.
4. Repeat for a total of three to five repetitions.

STANDING REACH AND SUPPORTED STANDING REACH

How Will This Exercise Help?

Strengthens ankles and calves to prevent turning of the ankles while walking. Improves your balance, posture, and coordination, and helps increase mobility. Helps to prevent and relieve leg cramps.

Special Notes

Stare at one spot on the wall in front of you to help keep your balance. If you can't reach over your head, just lift your arms as high as you can comfortably. If

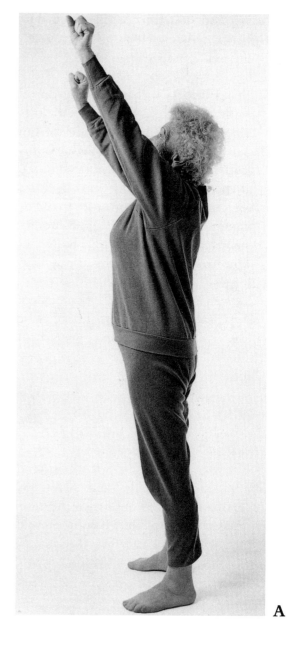

A

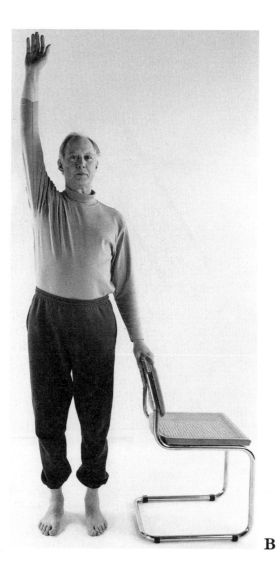

B

your balance is poor, do the Supported Standing Reach variation at first (see below).

1. Stand up straight and breathe gently in and out through your nose three times.
2. Stare at one spot on the wall or floor for balance and breathe out completely.
3. Breathe in and raise both your arms to the sides in a wide circle and overhead as high as possible without straining. Make fists and push up toward the ceiling (A). Hold your breath in and look up for a count of three.
4. Breathe out as you slowly lower your arms to your sides. Relax.
5. Repeat twice more.

Variations

If this exercise becomes too easy for you, come up on your toes when you breathe in and lift your arms. Hold for a count of three, then breathe out and come down on your heels while lowering your arms. This will greatly increase your stability and balance.

SUPPORTED STANDING REACH

1. Hold on to the back of the chair with one hand. Breathe out completely.
2. Breathe in as you lift the other arm over your head, make a fist, and push up toward the ceiling (B). Hold your breath for a count of three. Be sure to stare at one spot for balance. Breathe out and lower.
3. Repeat three times on each side.

SUPPORTED REACH ON TOES

1. Hold on to the back of the chair with one hand. Breathe out completely.
2. Breathe in as you lift the other arm, raise your heels, and come up on your toes. Make a fist and hold your breath in for a count of three. If possible, look up at your hand (C).
3. Repeat three times on each side.

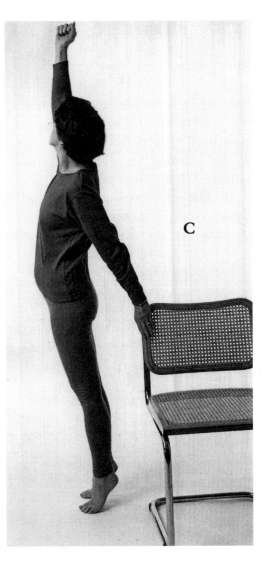

C

"Used to be I could only walk one way to the store, two blocks away; coming back I felt about dead. I'd have to stop and have someone come get me. Now I can go all the way to the grocery store and back because Yoga exercises have brought new strength into my legs. I can even stand up all the way through singing two hymns in church!"

—Ruby Allen (age 87)

TIP-TOE BALANCE

How Will This Exercise Help?

Increases limberness in the ankles, strengthens ankle and calf muscles, and improves balance and coordination. Improves breathing and posture. Helps to prevent and relieve leg cramps.

Special Notes

Remember to stare at one spot on the wall in front of you to help with balance.

1. Stand up straight and breathe in and out gently three times through your nose.
2. Breathe out completely. As you slowly breathe in, lift your heels, come up on your toes, and press your fists into your diaphragm (A). (Note: Press your fists into the soft area of the diaphragm just beneath the rib cage, not on the ribs themselves.)
3. Hold for a count of three, staring at one spot on the floor or wall for balance.
4. Slowly breathe out as you lower your heels to the floor and arms to your sides. Rest and relax.
5. Repeat twice more.

Variations

If you are frail, hold on to a support with one hand and press in on the diaphragm with one fist only (B).

"I do some of my balancing exercises while I wash dishes."

—Myrtis Weeks (age 81)

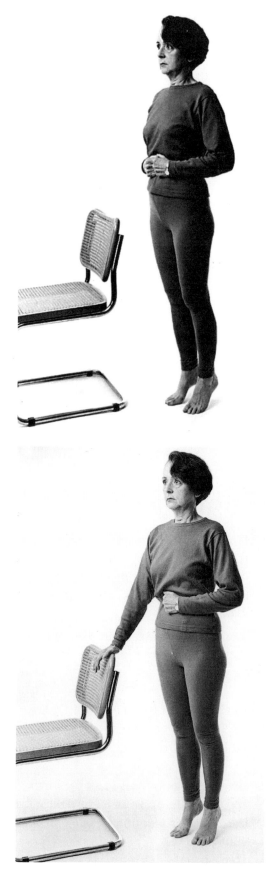

A

B

GENTLE FULL BENDS AND SUPPORTED FULL BEND

How Will This Exercise Help?

Increases limberness in the shoulders. Gives you a full body stretch, which strengthens the nervous and endocrine systems, improves circulation, and tones muscles. Improves heart function and balance.

Special Notes

Be sure not to do this exercise too quickly, like a toe-touch in calisthenics. All movements should be slow and gentle, coordinated with your breathing. If you have high blood pressure and your doctor has told you not to bend your head lower than your heart, bend only halfway down.

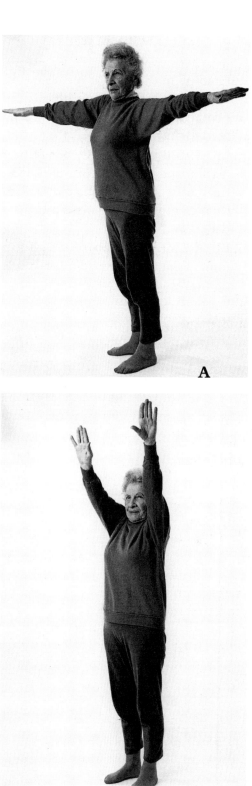

A

B

1. Stand up straight and breathe in and out three times through your nose.
2. Breathe in as you lift your arms out to the sides in a wide circle (A) and up overhead (B). Look up. Do not strain. Hold for a count of three.
3. Slowly breathe out as you bend forward from the waist, tucking your head. Reach as far forward toward the floor as you can without straining (C). Hold your breath out for a count of three.
4. Breathe in deeply as you come back up, lifting your arms out to the sides in another circle and overhead. Look up at your hands and hold for a count of three with your breath held in.
5. Breathe out and relax, arms to your sides. Repeat three to five times.

"I have more confidence in myself because I don't have to hang on to the chair when I do my balance exercises."
—Ruby Allen (age 87)

SUPPORTED FULL BEND

1. Hold on to the back of the chair with one hand.
2. Slowly breathe in as you lift your other arm to the side and up, reaching for the ceiling. Look up and hold for a count of three.
3. Breathe out as you gently bend from the hips, reaching forward and down in front toward the floor (D). Keep arm and knees straight. It doesn't matter how close to the floor you get. Hold for a count of three with your breath out.
4. Breathe in as you come back up to a standing position, raising your arm out to the side in a circle and up overhead again.
5. Rest and relax.
6. Repeat on the opposite side.

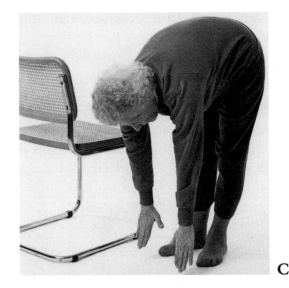

C

"Because of my physical limitation, good blood circulation is a must and I get such a beautiful feeling from the exercise— I can actually feel the circulation and more oxygen in my brain by stretching. After Yoga I tingle all over, as though I'm waking up. That's how I know when my circulation's improved."

—Dorothy Wild (age 69)

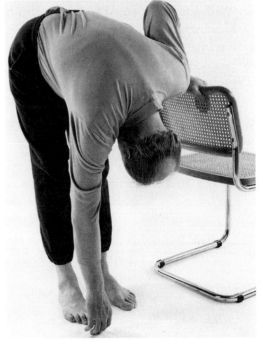

D

STANDING LEG LIFTS

How Will This Exercise Help?

Limbers the hip joint and strengthens the muscles of the hips and legs. Helps trim the fatty areas of buttocks and thighs. If you are recovering from an injury, this exercise will help you safely build strength in your back, legs, and hips. Improves heart function.

Special Notes

Be sure your support is sturdy and that you are standing on a nonskid surface. If you are afraid of falling, hold on to the chair back with both hands instead of one. Stare at one spot on the wall in front of you for balance.

Keep your torso upright at all times, especially during the rear leg lift, so you feel the movement in your hip joints.

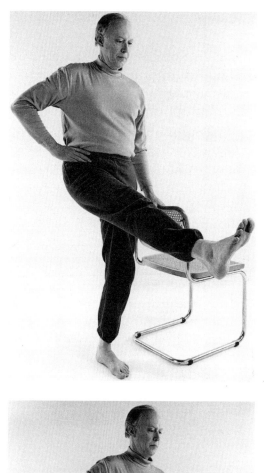

A

1. Stand up straight and to the right of a chair or railing. Hold tightly with your left hand. Place your right hand on your hip. Breathe in and out slowly three times, then breathe out completely.
2. Breathe in as you lift your right leg straight up in front as high as possible without bending your knee or straining (A). Hold the position and your breath for a count of three.
3. Breathe out and lower your leg. Shake it out.
4. Breathe in and lift your leg straight out to the side as far as possible without straining (B). Hold the position and your breath for a count of three.
5. Breathe out and lower your leg. Shake it out.
6. Breathe in and lift your right leg straight out in back as far as possible without bending your knee (C). Hold the position and your breath for a count of three.
7. Breathe out and lower your leg. Shake it out.
8. Repeat with your left leg.

B

Variations

If you have very weak leg and back muscles, begin by holding for a shorter count and slowly working to increase the time held.

> *"I suffer from arthritis. Not so much in my joints like some folks; mine's in the thick part of my thigh. At night it aches just like a toothache. I know it's Yoga that's made the difference because I'd go to the doctor and get shots and medicine, but it didn't go away. Since I started Yoga, it doesn't seem to bother me as much."*
>
> —Alberta Hendrix (age 71)

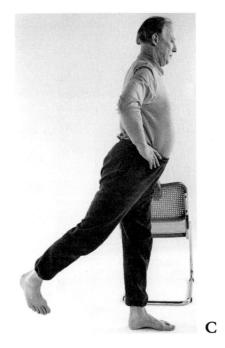

C

STANDING KNEE SQUEEZE

How Will This Exercise Help?

Helps develop balance and concentration. Strengthens the arms, shoulders, legs, and feet, and improves circulation and digestion. Improves heart function.

Special Notes

Do not attempt the more advanced version until you are confident in the supported version. If you have arthritis or other joint problems in your knees, grasp underneath the thigh near the knee instead.

1. Stand straight, holding on to a chair or railing with your right hand. Breathe gently in and out three times through your nose, then breathe out completely.
2. Breathe in deeply as you raise your left knee in front of you.
3. Hold your breath in and wrap your left arm around your knee. Gently squeeze the knee toward your chest (A). If possible, bend your head toward your knee slightly and try to put your forehead on your knee. Hold your breath in for a count of three.
4. Breathe out as you relax and lower your leg to the floor. Rest.
5. Repeat on the opposite side, rest, then repeat twice

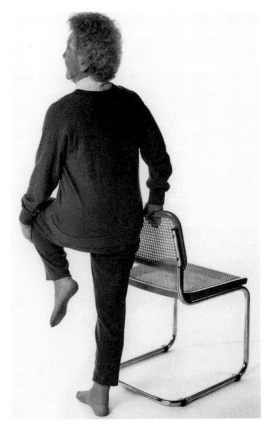

A

more on each side, alternating, for a total of three times on each leg.

Variation

When your strength and balance improve, try this exercise with both arms wrapped around the upraised knee (B).

"It feels good to get fresh blood up into my brains. I even think Yoga exercise has helped my hair to start growing back again. My mother's ninety-two, and the last time I saw her, she thought I was wearing a rug!"

—Gene Roy (age 62)

REAR ARM LIFT

How Will This Exercise Help?

Improves breathing capacity and heart function by stretching the muscles of the rib cage, chest, and upper back. Improves posture and helps to straighten rounded shoulders.

Special Notes

Since lifting your arms to the back is not a common movement, be careful not to strain when doing this exercise for the first time. It will help to massage your shoulders (see p. 73) before and after this exercise.

1. Stand erect, with hands clasped behind your back.
2. Breathe out completely.
3. Breathe in as you lift your arms up and away from your body, keeping your hands together. Try not to bend forward, and keep your head erect.
4. Hold your breath in for a count of three, then breathe out and relax, lowering your arms to your sides.
5. Repeat twice more.

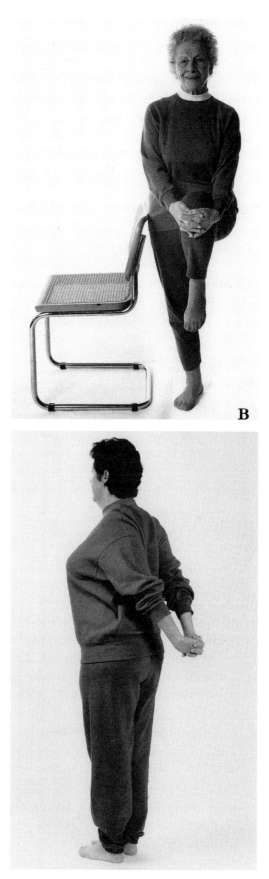

B

Variations

If you are very limber, you may try to straighten your elbows into a locked position so that the palms are pressed together in back. This is a difficult movement because it requires great limberness of the shoulders and upper back, but it greatly improves respiration and posture when practiced regularly.

TREE POSE

How Will This Exercise Help?

Develops concentration, poise, and balance. Strengthens your leg muscles and promotes a healthy, strong nervous system. Strengthens heart and lungs.

Special Notes

It's important in this exercise to try to relax your stomach and breathing muscles so you breathe normally throughout the exercise. Most people tend to hold their breath while trying to balance on one leg, even while supported, so constantly remind yourself to relax your breath. Do all movements slowly, step by step; don't try to leap to the full balance position all at once. Remember to stare at one spot on the wall or floor in front of you to help you balance.

Many people have trouble finding a comfortable place to rest their lifted foot on the opposite leg. Most people have success if they hook the foot just above the opposite knee joint to anchor it in place. If you remember to let your lifted leg relax, it will stay in place better. It also helps to do this exercise in bare feet.

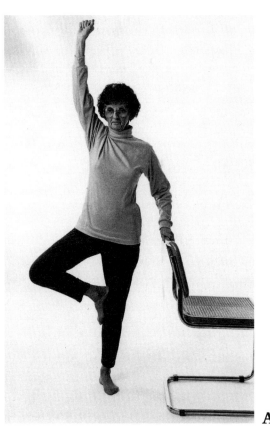

A

1. Stand straight, holding on to the back of a sturdy chair with your left hand for support. Stare at one spot on the wall or floor for balance. Gently breathe in and out three times.
2. Breathe normally as you lift your right foot and place it on the inside of your left leg, as high up as you can. Let your right leg relax so it will stay in place better.
3. When you feel steady, breathe in as you slowly lift

your right arm overhead (A). Keep staring at one spot. Hold your breath in for a count of three.

4. Relax, breathe out, and lower your arm and leg.
5. Repeat on the opposite side.

Variations

When you are confident with this exercise, try lifting both arms overhead in Step 4 (B). Remember to stare at one spot for balance.

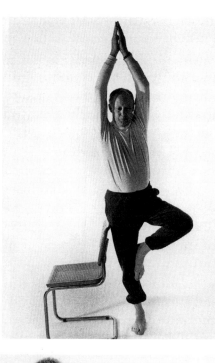

B

"I can stand on one foot and put on my socks now instead of holding on to a chair for balance. And I can do that Tree Pose with my foot way up on my leg. At sixty-four, I think that's quite an accomplishment!"

—Helen Gould (age 64)

REAR LEG LIFTS AND SUPER BALANCE POSE

How Will This Exercise Help?

Strengthens legs, hips, and back muscles, limbers hip joints, improves balance and concentration, and improves circulation to the extremities. Increases confidence in walking and other activities. Strengthens heart and lungs.

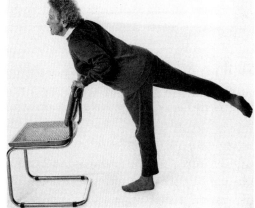

A

1. Stand facing the back of your chair and hold on with both hands. Be sure you have enough room in back of you to lift your leg.
2. Step back from the chair and lean forward slightly.
3. Breathe out completely. Breathe in and slowly lift your right leg in back as high as you can without strain (A). Try to lift your back leg parallel to the floor—but without straining. Keep both legs straight but do not lock your knees. Hold your breath in for a count of three.
4. Breathe out and lower your leg. Rest.
5. Repeat with the left leg, then twice more on each side, alternating.

Now try the Super Balance Pose:

1. Holding on to the chair with both hands as above, back away from the chair and lean forward.

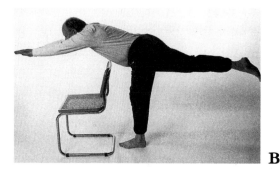

B

2. Breathe normally—don't hold your breath.

3. Slowly lift your right leg in back, keeping both legs straight.

4. Hold the position, breathing normally, and slowly loosen your grip on the chair. Do not let go completely! If you feel really steady, you can straighten your arms just above the chair (B), but be ready to grab hold again immediately if you feel unsteady. Look forward across your outstretched hands. Remember to keep breathing normally.

5. Grasp the chair again, lower your leg, and relax. Rest.

6. Repeat with the left leg.

"It's helped me in particular to be able to sweep the floor better. I didn't very often sweep or vacuum the floor before I started this Yoga exercise. Now I can get right down to plug in the vacuum and then I can get right back up. Isn't that something?"

—Ada Duffy (age 77)

SIMPLE ALTERNATE TRIANGLE

How Will This Exercise Help?

Stretches back of legs and lower back. Improves limberness of hips, shoulders, and spine. Stimulates circulation throughout the body, eyes, and brain. May help relieve depression. Helps improve heart and lung function.

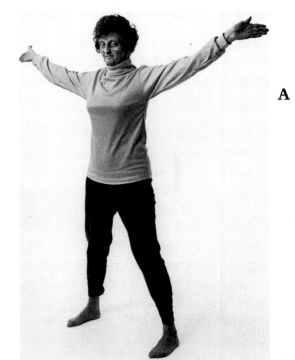

A

Special Notes

Be sure not to strain. If you notice any pain or stiffness the next day, you are bending too far forward. If you have high blood pressure and your doctor has told you not to put your head lower than your heart, bend only halfway down in Step 3.

1. Stand with your feet apart a comfortable distance and toes pointed forward.

2. Breathe in completely as you lift your arms and open them wide to the sides to shoulder height (A).

3. Breathe out as you slowly bend toward one leg and grasp your leg with both hands as far down the leg as

you can comfortably. Pull gently by bending your elbows (B). Hold your breath out for a count of three.

4. Breathe in and stand up, opening your arms out again.
5. Repeat on the opposite side. Rest.
6. Repeat twice more to each leg, alternating sides.

Variations

If you are unsure of your balance, do this exercise facing the back of a sturdy chair. Hold on with your right hand while you bend toward the left leg, and vice versa.

"My forward-bending exercises are a must every day. They do a lot for my circulation. When I bend over I can actually feel the fresh blood rushing down into my fingertips and back up into my arms."

—Josephine Vidmar (age 70)

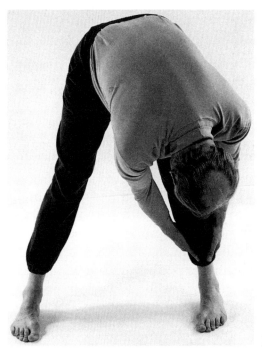

B

CHAPTER 7

Exercises for Bed or Floor

"Why, I can even get down on the floor now. I get right down and right back up again. I could never do that before. I used to be terribly afraid of getting down on the floor, but no more—no sirree!"

—Ada Duffy (age 77)

This chapter includes one of the most important techniques that Easy Does It Yoga has to offer: how to get down on the floor and back up again. If you have trouble doing this, you must be familiar with the feelings of frustration that come from not being able to perform such routine tasks as cleaning a bottom shelf or picking up the newspaper from the floor. Our technique is very simple, and I urge you to learn it as soon as possible. Practicing will free you from the fear that one day you will fall and have to wait, helpless, until someone can help you get up again. We begin the chapter with some preparatory exercises to practice first in case you need to develop strength in your arms and legs.

Once you have mastered this technique, you can begin to practice some of the Easy Does It Yoga exercises in this section that are done on the floor. (Remember that many of these can also be done in bed; a special symbol 🛏 indicates these.) Start with the seated positions and slowly work into the lying-down positions. To move from a seated to a lying-down position, first rest on one elbow, supporting your weight with your opposite hand, and then slowly lower yourself onto your back. To get back up to a seated position, roll to one side, place one hand in back for support, roll up on one elbow, then push up to a seated position.

Floor exercises will be more comfortable if you practice on a soft foam mat or a folded blanket.

Most of the floor exercises can also be practiced in bed on a firm mattress. Consider doing a few exercises first thing in the morning before you get out of bed to help work through normal morning stiffness.

LAZY KNEE BENDS

How Will This Exercise Help?

Strengthens knees and ankles, and builds confidence, in preparation for getting down on the floor without strain.

Special Notes

Be sure to keep your torso straight while bending your knees; otherwise your back is getting the exercise instead of your legs.

1. There are two parts to this exercise. To warm up, just hold on to a chair with both hands and slowly bend your knees and then straighten them—bend just a few inches at first (A). Keep your feet flat on the floor. Breathe normally throughout. Repeat several times.
2. Stand away from the chair, reach down, and place your hands firmly on your knees.
3. Gently bend and straighten your knees as before, keeping your feet flat. Don't bend too far. Keep your hands on your knees for support.

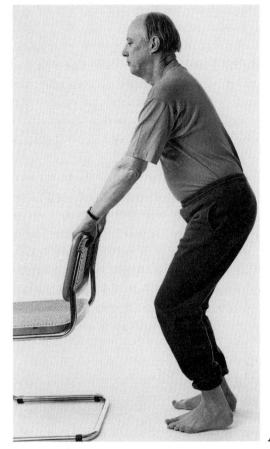

A

LEG AND ARM STRENGTHENERS

How Will This Exercise Help?

Builds upper arm and shoulder strength, and improves hand grip, to help in the technique of getting down to the floor and back up safely.

Special Notes

For the quickest results, practice both variations of this exercise at home several times a day.

Many students have a tendency to place their feet away from the chair, making it harder to bend the knees and causing more strain on the arms. One foot should always be close to the front chair leg; when the front

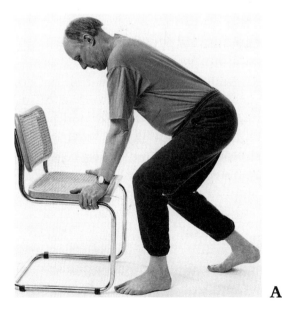

A

knee bends, the knee should extend slightly out to one side, not straight forward into the chair.

As you repeat this exercise every day, gradually bend further down until you can rest one knee on the floor and push yourself back up to a standing position, using your arms. You will then be ready to move on to the actual technique of getting down to the floor. Use a foam pad under your knees to prevent discomfort.

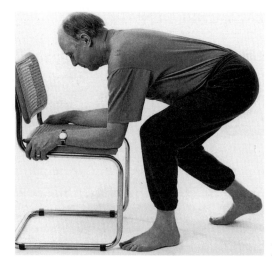

B

1. Stand facing your chair. Lean forward and grasp the sides of the chair seat firmly with both hands.
2. Place your left foot near the left front leg of the chair, and your right foot behind you.
3. Leaning on your hands, slowly bend your knees (A), keeping your weight on your hands, and then use your hands to push yourself back up. Bend as far as you can and still be able to straighten up again.
4. Repeat with the right foot forward and left foot back.

Variations

When you become stronger, do the same exercise with your forearms resting on the seat of the chair and elbows bent (B).

GETTING DOWN ON THE FLOOR

How Will This Exercise Help?

Knowing how to get down on the floor and back up safely will improve your confidence and self-esteem by increasing your feelings of independence. This technique also builds physical strength and stamina, which contribute to feelings of well-being.

Special Notes

Give yourself a period of several weeks to learn this exercise completely, depending on how often you practice it and how frail you are to begin with. Be sure to use a sturdy chair on a carpet or other nonskid surface.

If you have one knee with arthritis or other joint

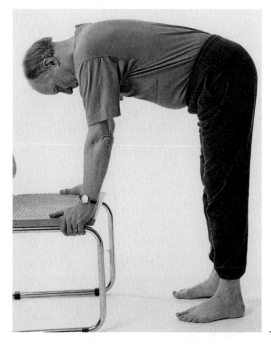

A

problems that would make putting weight on the joint painful, make sure that you bend with the other (good) knee toward the floor. A foam rubber pad in front of the chair on the floor will also help to protect your knees.

If you have chronic, painful knee joint problems affecting both knees, or if you have very weak arms, it may take some time for you to develop the strength to do this exercise safely. In these cases, practice the preparatory exercises (Lazy Knee Bends, and Leg and Arm Strengtheners) first for several days or weeks to build strength in your arms and legs and to practice the coordination of the various movements needed in this technique.

1. Stand facing the front of a sturdy chair, bend at the waist, and grasp the outside edges of the chair seat firmly (A).
2. Place your left foot near the front left chair leg and your right foot slightly behind you.
3. Supporting yourself on your hands, bend your knees and slowly lower your left knee toward the floor (B). (Remember, if you have problems with your left knee, reverse positions and bend your right knee down instead.)
4. Continuing to hold on to the chair seat for support, slowly lower your right knee to the floor (C).
5. Hold on to the chair with your right hand and carefully place your left hand on the floor near your left hip (D).
6. Shifting your weight to your left arm, carefully bring your right hand down to the floor on your left side so you are leaning on both hands (E).
7. Supporting your weight on both hands, slowly lower your hips toward the floor near your left hand (F).
8. Bring your hands around to support you in back and slowly straighten your right leg (G).
9. Unfold your left leg so you are sitting with both legs outstretched, leaning on your hands (H). Now you are ready to do any of the floor exercises in this chapter.

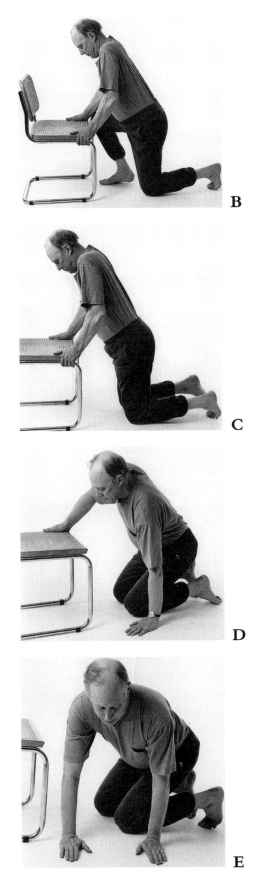

B

C

D

E

To Get Up From the Floor

1. Starting from a seated position with legs outstretched (H), bend both knees and let your legs bend toward the right.
2. Place both hands next to your right hip (F).
3. Carefully push yourself up on your hands and knees, using your arms (E).
4. Walk on all fours over to a sturdy chair.
5. Lift your right hand and grasp the side of the chair seat firmly (D), then grasp the other side of the chair seat with your left hand.
6. Holding on firmly to the chair seat, move forward on your knees so you are close to the chair. Tuck your toes under (C).
7. Carefully raise your right foot and place it flat on the floor (B).
8. Putting your weight on your arms, push yourself up so you are standing on both feet (A). (Some of you may have more success by resting your forearms instead of your hands on the chair in this step.)
9. Slowly stand up.

"That way of getting up and down is really great. My friends wanted to know how to do it, so I said, 'I'll show you how easy it is. It's just a matter of putting your legs and hands in the right place!' I showed them how, and they said, 'Well, there's nothing to it! That's really easy!' And you come up the same way you went down. It's great!"

—Myrtis Weeks (age 81)

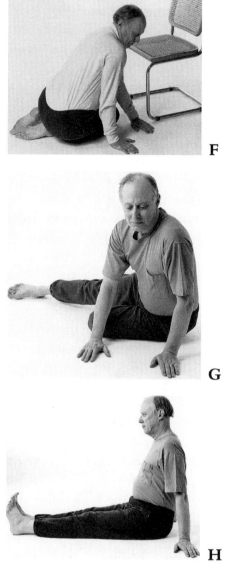

F

G

H

SUN POSE STRETCH

How Will This Exercise Help?

This exercise is a nonstrenuous warm-up that prepares you for the Seated Sun Pose by gently stretching and strengthening the lower back. Helps prevent sciatica, improves digestion, and stimulates circulation in vital organs. Improves heart and lung function. Helps straighten a hunched back by lengthening the spine.

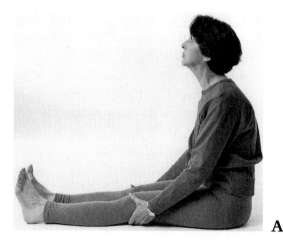

A

Special Notes

If you have lower back problems, be very careful not to stretch forward too far in this exercise to avoid straining the muscles of your lower back.

1. Sit straight with legs outstretched. Your legs should be very straight, with the backs of your knees touching the floor if possible. Place your hands under your legs near your knees.
2. Take in a deep breath as you straighten your back, look up, and pull your upper body slightly toward your legs by bending your elbows (A). Hold your breath and the position for a count of three.
3. Breathe out as you round your back and tuck your head forward, pulling your chin into your throat (B). Hold your breath out for a count of three.
4. Breathe in and return to position (A).
5. Repeat twice more.

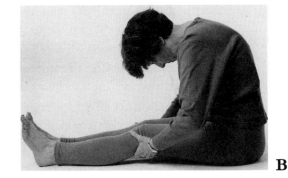

B

SEATED SUN POSE

How Will This Exercise Help?

Strengthens abdominal muscles, improves digestion and breathing, stretches and strengthens legs and spine. May help prevent sciatica. Improves heart and lung function. Reduces a large stomach.

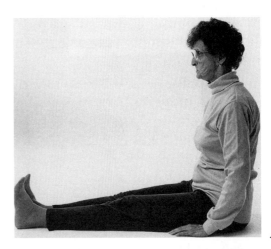

A

Special Notes

To help prevent cramps, rest frequently and relax all your limbs. At Step 5, be sure to pull by bending your arms, not by pushing with your lower back. If you have lower back problems, do not pull at all, but simply bend forward over your legs as far as you can comfortably.

Note that this exercise uses two complete breath cycles. Be sure to complete the pose (arms to sides: Step 7 below) and rest for at least 30 seconds before repeating the exercise.

1. Sit straight with legs outstretched (A). Breathe in and out three times through your nose.

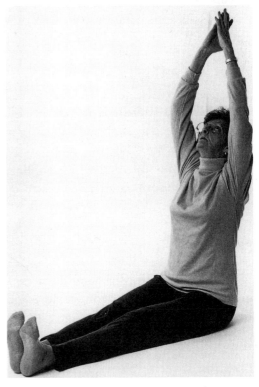

B

2. Start with Foot Flaps: Pull your toes back toward your face and then push them forward, several times.

3. Next, do Ankle Rotations: Rotate both ankles to the right three times, then to the left three times, then rotate ankles toward each other three times, then away from each other three times. Return your feet to the pointed-back position for the Seated Sun Pose.

4. Breathe out completely. Breathe in as you raise your arms in a wide circle and over your head. Look up and hold your breath for a count of three (B).

5. Breathe out as you tuck your head and bend forward over your legs. Grasp firmly underneath your legs and bend your elbows, pulling your upper body toward your legs (C). Hold your breath out for a count of three.

6. Release and start to breathe in as you raise your arms in another wide circle overhead (B). Look up.

7. Breathe out and relax, arms to sides. Rest for about 30 seconds.

8. Repeat twice more.

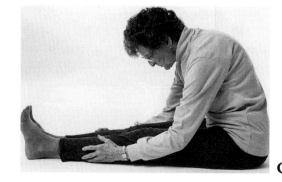

C

Variations

If you are bedridden, you can do the Foot Flaps and Ankle Rotations lying on your back.

EASY ALTERNATE SUN POSE

How Will This Exercise Help?

This exercise stretches the groin muscles and limbers the knee joints in addition to all the benefits of the Seated Sun Pose.

Special Notes

If you have arthritic or painful knees, bend your knee only as far as you can comfortably and place a pillow under your bent knee. Massage your knees before and after this exercise (see p. 74).

At Step 3, be sure to pull by bending your arms, not by pushing with your lower back. If you have lower

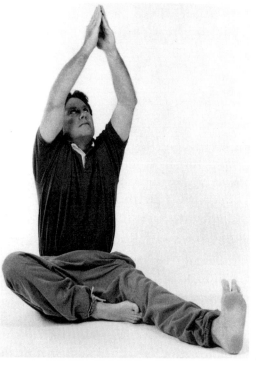

A

back problems, do not pull at all, but simply bend forward over your legs as far as you can do so comfortably.

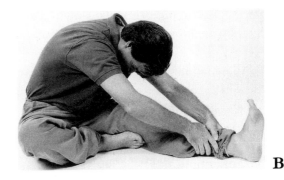

B

1. Sit straight with legs together. Bend your right leg and place your right foot flat as high up on the inside of your left leg as you can without straining. Your left leg should be straight, with the toes of your left foot pointed back toward your face. Breathe in and out three times through your nose.
2. Breathe out completely, then breathe in as you raise your arms in a wide circle to the sides and overhead. Look up (A) and hold your breath for a count of three.
3. Breathe out as you tuck your head and bend forward over your left leg, keeping the toes of your left leg flexed toward your face. Grasp firmly underneath your leg and bend your elbows, pulling your upper body toward your leg (B). Hold your breath for a count of three.
4. Release and breathe in deeply as you raise your arms in another wide circle overhead. Look up and hold your breath for a count of three.
5. Breathe out and relax, bringing your arms slowly down to your sides. Rest for at least 30 seconds.
6. Repeat twice more. Straighten the leg and massage the knee.
7. Repeat three times on opposite side.

GENTLE TWIST

How Will This Exercise Help?

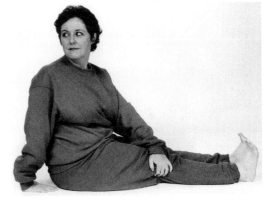

Improves flexibility of the spine and increases circulation to the brain. Helps in daily activities such as being able to turn around while backing up a car. Also strengthens shoulder and arm muscles, and improves memory, eyesight, heart function, and breathing.

Special Notes

Be sure to keep your spine as straight as possible while turning in order to get a true sideways twist. The hand in back should be as close to your body as possible, fingers pointed in. When you twist back, exercise your eyes by looking as far back as you can.

1. Sit straight with legs together, pointed front. Toes should be pointed toward the ceiling. Breathe in and out three times through your nose.
2. Place your right hand across your left thigh and place your left hand in back of you, palm down, fingers pointing in toward your back. Place the hand as close to your body as you can.
3. Sit up straight and look forward. Breathe in completely.
4. Breathe out as you slowly turn and look back over your left shoulder. Use your arms to pull and push yourself around as far as you can without straining.
5. Look at a spot on the wall at eye level with your eyes as far left as you can see and hold your breath out for a count of three.
6. Breathe in, release, and turn back to the front. Relax.
7. Repeat on the other side.

SPINE TWIST

How Will This Exercise Help?

Improves flexibility of the spine and increases circulation to the brain. Helps in daily activities such as being able to turn around while backing up a car. Also strengthens shoulder and arm muscles, and improves memory, eyesight, heart function, and breathing.

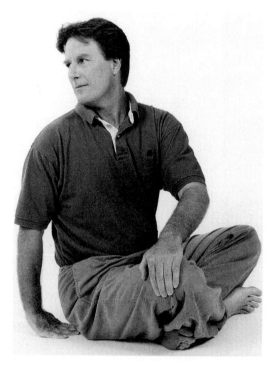

Special Notes

Be sure to keep your spine as straight as possible while turning in order to get a true sideways twist. The hand in back should be as close to your body as possible, fingers pointed in. When you twist back, exercise your eyes by looking as far back as you can.

1. Sit in a cross-legged position as in the photo. Breathe in and out three times.
2. Place your right hand on your left knee and place your left hand in back of you, palm down, fingers pointed in toward your back.

3. Straighten your back and breathe in, then breathe out as you gently turn toward the left, pushing and pulling slightly with both hands to stretch as far as you can without straining. Look as far to the left as you can and fix your gaze on a spot on the wall just above eye level.
4. Hold your breath out for a count of three, then breathe in, turn forward, and relax.
5. Repeat on the opposite side. Rest and relax.
6. Repeat twice more on each side, alternating.

ALTERNATE TORTOISE STRETCH

How Will This Exercise Help?

Improves circulation to the pelvic region, stretches nerves and muscles in the legs and ankles, limbers the lower back, and helps prevent prostate and urinary problems due to poor circulation. Helps improve memory.

Special Notes

If you have lower back or sciatica problems, be very careful when bending forward and reach down only as far as your knees at first.

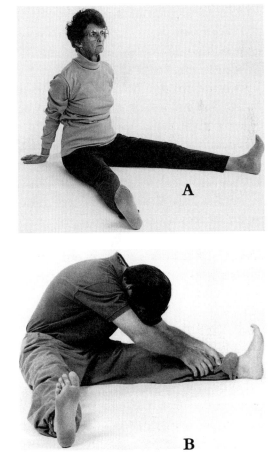

1. Sit straight and separate your legs as far as you can. Your toes should be pointed toward the ceiling (A). Breathe in and out three times.
2. Breathe out completely, then breathe in deeply as you raise your arms in a circle to the sides and overhead. Look up and hold your breath in for a count of three.
3. Breathe out as you bend toward your left leg, tucking your chin into your throat. Grasp your left leg firmly and bend your elbows to pull your upper body gently toward your leg (B). Do not strain! Hold your breath out for a count of three.
4. Release your leg, breathe in deeply, and come back up, bringing your arms in another wide circle to the sides and overhead. Look up and hold your breath for a count of three.
5. Breathe out and lower your arms. Rest for at least 30 seconds, then repeat to the right side. Repeat twice more on each side, alternating.

SUPER STRENGTHENING REACH

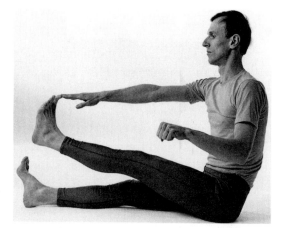

How Will This Exercise Help?

Strengthens abdominal muscles, improves digestion and breathing, stretches and strengthens hips, legs, and spine. May help prevent sciatica. Improves heart and lung function. Reduces a large stomach.

Special Notes

This exercise requires a bit more strength than other "toe-touching" exercises, especially in your lower back. We do not suggest this exercise for people with lower back problems. Be sure not to strain to reach your toes at first. You can also practice this exercise sitting in the bathtub or on the steps of a shallow pool; the buoyancy of the water will make the exercise a little easier on your back.

1. Sit straight, with legs outstretched in front of you. Breathe in and out three times.
2. Point your toes back toward your face without bending your knees, and place both hands on top of your thighs.
3. Breathe in and hold your breath as you lift your left leg and reach out toward your left toes with your right hand (opposites). Hold for a count of three. Breathe out and relax back to your starting position.
4. Repeat with left hand and right leg.
5. Rest at least 30 seconds, breathing normally.
6. If you are strong enough, repeat twice more on each side, alternating.
7. Lean back on your hands and rest, breathing gently, until you are completely relaxed.

KNEE SQUEEZE

How Will This Exercise Help?

Limbers the back and hips, relieves lower back tension, strengthens abdominal muscles, and improves the function of the heart, lungs, and digestive organs.

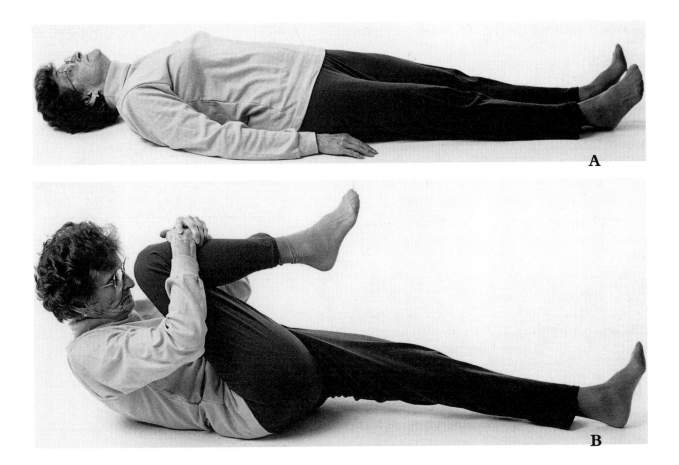

A

B

Special Notes

If you have lower back problems, do this exercise with your knees bent and feet flat on the floor several inches apart.

Note that in this exercise, unlike most others in this book, the breath is held *in* as the body is compressed; this is essential for the effectiveness of the exercise as it provides both inner and outer pressure on the lungs and other internal organs.

1. Lie on your back with arms at your sides and legs together (A). Breathe in and out three times.
2. Breathe out completely.
3. Breathe in as you bend your right knee and grasp it with both hands, bringing it in toward your chest, then squeeze your knee to your chest and lift your forehead up toward your knee (B). Hold your breath in for a count of three.
4. Relax and breathe out as you lower your head, arms, and legs down to the floor. Rest a few seconds, then

repeat with the left leg. Repeat twice more on each side, alternating.

Variations

Double Knee Squeeze: Start with both legs bent and feet flat on the floor about 18 inches apart. Breathe in and hold your breath in as you lift both knees, squeezing them to your chest with both arms and lifting your forehead toward your knees (C). Breathe out and return your feet to the floor as in your starting position.

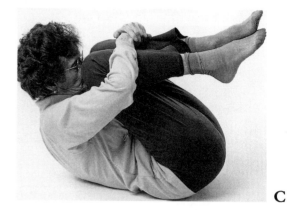

C

> *"I was in the hospital a year ago for some back trouble and I couldn't do some of the floor exercises. So I do a lot of those bed exercises. I always do these Knee Squeezes every morning before getting out of bed."*
> —Pauline Moody (age 73)

EASY BRIDGE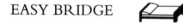

How Will This Exercise Help?

Improves functioning of thyroid and entire glandular system, relieves lower back pain and fatigue, improves complexion and strengthens eyes by bringing circulation to the head, and can help to relieve bedsores. Improves heart function.

Special Notes

This exercise should be done as a half lift, not a full arched bridge, which puts much more stress on the back of the neck.

1. Lie on your back and bend your knees. Place your feet flat on the floor (or bed) several inches apart, and bring them as close to your hips as possible. Lay your arms palms down at your sides (A). Breathe in and out three times through your nose.
2. Breathe out completely. Relax your shoulders.
3. Breathe in slowly as you raise your hips off the floor, curling your lower spine up to your waist. Your waist

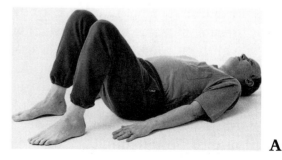

A

should remain on the floor (B). Hold your breath and this position for a count of three.

4. Breathe out as you slowly lower your hips to the floor. Relax fully, stretching out your legs.
5. Return your legs to the bent position and repeat the exercise twice more.

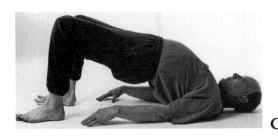

B

Variations

When you get stronger, and if you have no neck problems, you may try a full arched pose: Your hips are raised higher and your entire spine arched as much as possible so that your chin is tucked into your chest (C). In this version, your entire back is lifted off the floor and your weight shifts to the back of your neck; you should not do this variation if you have any disk problems in your neck. Use the same breath pattern as above.

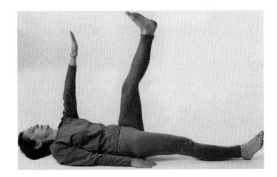

C

ALTERNATE TOE TOUCH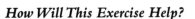

How Will This Exercise Help?

Stretches and strengthens the muscles and joints of the legs, hips, and lower back; helps relieve sciatica. Improves heart and lung function. Helps prevent a hunched back. Builds stamina.

Special Notes

Both knees should remain straight, even if it means you cannot touch your toe at first.

1. Lie on your back with your legs straight, right arm over your head, and left arm at your side. Breathe in and out three times through your nose.
2. Breathe out completely, then breathe in deeply as you lift your right arm and right leg simultaneously. Reach toward your toe, but keep your shoulders on the floor. Don't bend your knees—it's more important to keep your knees straight than to touch your toe. Hold your breath in for a count of three.
3. Breathe out and relax, bringing your right arm down to the floor over your head.

4. Now bring your right arm by your side and lift the left arm over your head to do the exercise on the opposite side. Repeat twice more on each side, alternating.

Variations

If you have very weak hip and leg muscles, you may do this exercise with your knees bent and feet flat on the floor. Use the same breath pattern, and keep the leg bent as you lift it, reaching for your raised knee instead of your toes.

> *"I used to have burning pains, like the size of a fist, in my back. I strengthened my back, and now I don't have them anymore. It sure feels a whole lot better, believe me."*
> —Gene Roy (age 62)

LOWER BACK STRETCH

How Will This Exercise Help?

Improves functioning of internal organs. Improves circulation. Strengthens and limbers the shoulders, back, and hip joints. Helps to trim the waistline.

Special Notes

If you have spinal disk problems in your lower back, be very careful with this exercise and be sure to check with your physician before you try it.

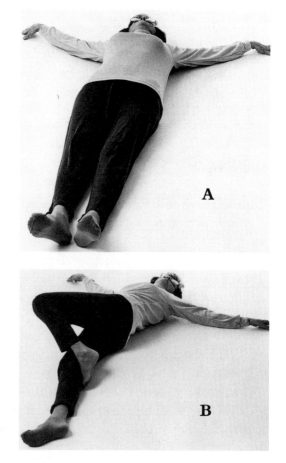

1. Lie on your back with your legs together and arms stretched out to the sides, palms down (A). Breathe in and out three times through your nose.
2. Breathe out, then breathe in as you bend your left leg and touch your left toe next to your right knee.
3. Breathe out as you bend your left leg to the right over your right leg, keeping your left toe touching your right knee. Continue moving your left leg across your body as far as possible without straining (B). This will twist your hips to the right, pulling strongly on your

waist and lower back. Keep your shoulders and arms on the floor and keep your right leg straight.

4. Hold your breath out in this position for a count of three.
5. Breathe in as you roll back, lift your left knee up, and straighten your leg toward the ceiling.
6. Breathe out as you return the leg to the floor. Rest at least 30 seconds, then repeat on the other side.

EASY COBRA LIFT

How Will This Exercise Help?

Limbers and strengthens the entire spinal column and back muscles. Strengthens upper back and shoulders. Improves breathing and eyesight. Activates sexual function.

Special Notes

If you have spinal disk problems, do not do this exercise unless you have permission from your doctor. Be sure to begin this exercise in the correct position, with head and upper body relaxed.

1. Lie on your stomach and raise your body on your elbows, with the elbows close in to your body. Position your arms so that your elbows and shoulders are in a straight line up and down. Place your hands palms down in front of you. Let your forehead relax toward the floor and relax your shoulders (A).
2. Breathe out completely, then breathe in deeply as you slowly lift your head and stretch up and back without lifting your elbows off the floor. Look up

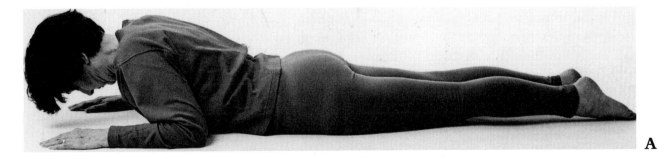

A

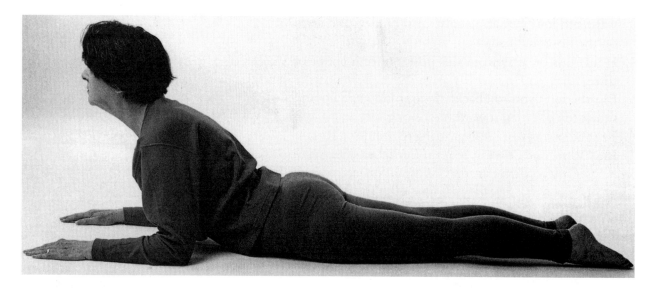

B

toward your forehead (B) and hold your breath in for a count of three.

3. Breathe out and slowly drop your forehead toward the floor and relax. Rest for at least 30 seconds, then repeat twice more.

Variation

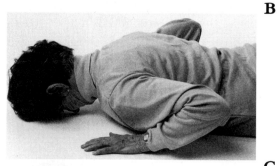

C

When you are stronger, you can try the full Cobra Pose: Lie on your stomach with your hands on the floor palms down next to your armpits (your elbows will be raised) (C). Place your forehead on the floor and relax your shoulders. Proceed as above, Steps 2 (D) and 3.

BACK STRENGTHENERS

How Will This Exercise Help?

D

Strengthens both sides of the back evenly. Stimulates circulation throughout the extremities and strengthens arms, shoulders, hips, and thighs. Improves heart, lung, and sexual function. Builds stamina. Improves posture, helping to prevent a hunched back.

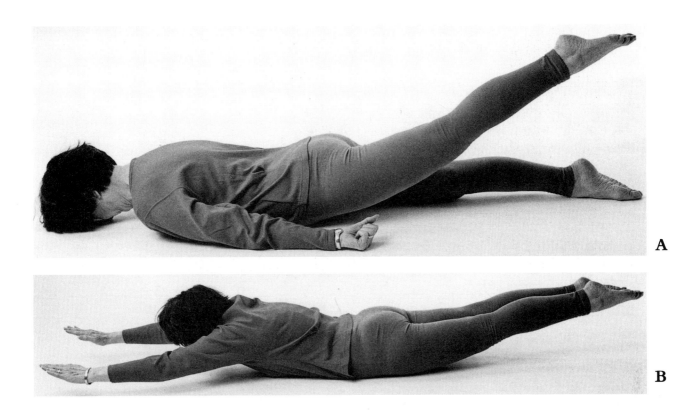

A

B

Special Notes

It is more important to keep your legs straight while lifting than to lift them high. If your legs are weak, you may be able to lift only an inch or two at first; with daily practice, you will build more strength very quickly.

1. Lie on your stomach with your forehead on the floor and arms at your sides. Breathe in and out three times through your nose.
2. Breathe out completely. Breathe in as you lift your left leg in back, keeping it straight (A). Hold your breath in for a count of three, maintaining the position.
3. Breathe out and lower the leg. Rest for at least 30 seconds.
4. Repeat with the right leg.
5. Repeat twice more on each side, alternating.
6. After resting for at least 30 seconds, stretch your arms in front of you and place your forehead on the floor.
7. Breathe out completely, then breathe in as you lift arms, head, and legs, keeping them straight (B). Look up and hold for a count of three.

8. Breathe out and lower to the floor. Relax and rest for at least 30 seconds, then repeat twice more.

"I used to have a pillow behind my back to drive my car. After I had practiced Yoga for some time my wife asked one day, 'Hey, where's your pillow?' I answered, 'What pillow? I don't need it anymore.' My back is much stronger now."

—Gene Roy (age 62)

ALL-FOURS LIFT

How Will This Exercise Help?

Strengthens shoulders, back, and hip joints; improves balance and posture. Helps prevent a hunched back.

Special Notes

To help with balance, stare at one spot on the floor in front of you as you do the exercise. In Step 7, remember to lift the *opposite* arm and leg. If you have lower back problems, do not hold at the top in Steps 2 and 7.

1. Come up to your hands and knees and look straight ahead. Breathe in and out three times through your nose.
2. Breathe out completely, then breathe in as you straighten your left leg and lift it up in back as high as you can (A). Hold your breath in for a count of three.
3. Breathe out and lower your leg. Rest.
4. Repeat with the right leg.
5. Repeat twice more on each leg, alternating.
6. After a rest, come back to your starting position. Breathe out.
7. Breathe in and slowly lift your *right* arm and your *left* leg (opposites) (B). Stare at one spot on the wall for balance. Hold your breath in for a count of three, maintaining the position.
8. Breathe out and lower your arm and leg to your starting position. Rest, then repeat on the opposite side.

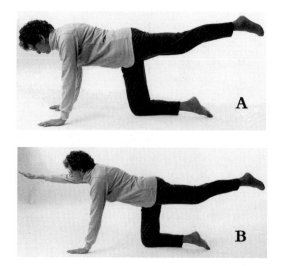

Variation

When your balance has improved, try lifting the arm and leg on the same side of your body, with the same breath pattern as above. This is much more difficult, so be sure to steady yourself by staring at one spot.

BABY POSE

How Will This Exercise Help?

Relieves fatigue. Improves circulation throughout the internal organs and brings fresh blood and oxygen to the brain. Improves eyesight, breathing, and heart function. Limbers the lower back, hips, knees, and feet. Improves digestion.

Special Notes

Never come up quickly from this position; blood draining from your head could cause feelings of faintness. Many students find this position very restful. Practice it at home as often as you wish.

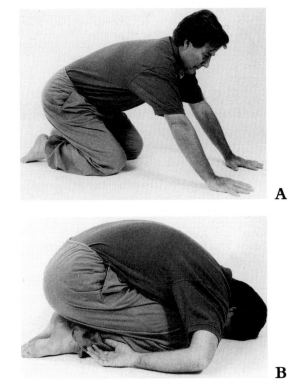

1. From a hands-and-knees position, be sure your toes are uncurled so that the tops of your feet rest against the floor. Keeping your hands on the floor, slowly sit back as far as possible (A). Ideally, your hips should rest on your heels. If you have arthritic knees, substitute the Folded Pose (see p. 84).
2. Bend forward so that your head rests on the floor in front of your knees. If that position is comfortable, bring your arms down to your sides with the elbows bent so they rest on the floor (B). Try to relax your whole body so that you go limp—just like a sack of potatoes. Especially relax the back of your neck. It is more important to keep your hips on your heels as you bend forward than to put your head on the floor; this increases the compression.
3. Breathe gently and rest for 15 seconds to a minute or more.
4. Return to a sitting position very slowly, pushing up with your hands.

Variations

If you are overweight, or feel uncomfortable when blood rushes to your head, you can rest your head on folded arms in front of your knees (C).

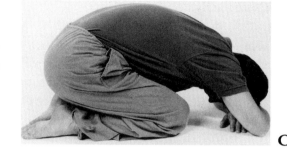

C

SHOULDER STAND PREPARATION

How Will This Exercise Help?

Stimulates the thyroid and parathyroid glands. Improves circulation, eyesight, memory, and breathing. Removes fatigue. Improves heart and sexual functions. Strengthens the legs and back in preparation for the Shoulder Stand. This is a lovely rest position that you can use any time to help remove fatigue.

Special Notes

Do not do this exercise if you have neck problems. Substitute the Easy Bridge (see p. 118) instead. If you have heart disease or high blood pressure, check with your doctor before trying this exercise. Practice on a soft foam mat or soft carpet to minimize discomfort on the back of your neck. Be sure the chair you use for support is stable and won't slip or skid.

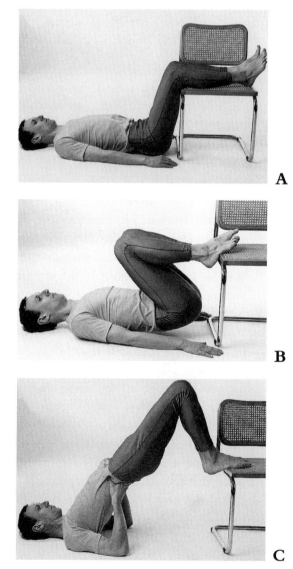

A

B

C

1. Lie down near a sturdy chair with your calves resting on the seat of the chair and your hips as close to the chair as possible (A).
2. Bring your legs back so your heels are resting on the edge of the chair seat (B).
3. Breathe out completely. Then, supporting your lower back with your hands, push your feet against the chair and breathe in as you lift your body up and your weight shifts to your shoulders and the back of your neck (C). Hold your breath in for a count of three.
4. Breathe out as you release and lower down carefully. Rest.

INVERTED REST POSE

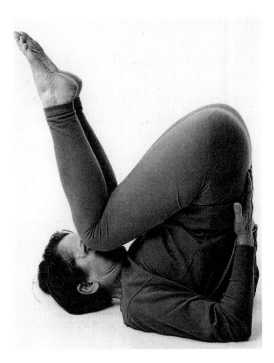

How Will This Exercise Help?

Tones the entire glandular system by stimulating the thyroid and parathyroid. Improves eyesight, breathing, and circulation. Removes fatigue.

Special Notes

This exercise should not be done by anyone with neck problems; substitute the Easy Bridge (p. 118) instead. If you have high blood pressure or heart disease, check with your doctor before trying this exercise.

Be sure to support your back properly in Step 3. Practice on a foam mat or soft carpet to minimize discomfort on the back of your neck.

1. Sit on the floor your with knees drawn up to your chest and arms wrapped around your knees. Keep your back rounded and your chin tucked into your throat.
2. Gently roll back and forth a few times, rolling onto your upper back and then forward to a sitting position.
3. Roll back on your upper back, keeping your knees bent toward your forehead, and immediately support your lower back with both hands, resting your elbows on the floor. Keep your knees bent toward your forehead at all times. Hold, breathing normally, for several seconds.
4. Release and gently roll forward to a sitting position, then lie on your back, keeping your knees bent and feet flat on the floor, and rest for at least one minute.

Variation

If you are afraid to roll back, or are very stiff, you can lie on your back with your hips pressed close to a chair or bed and your legs resting on top of the chair seat or the bed. Rest often like this to get used to the position, and soon you will be able to try the Inverted Rest Pose as described above.

SHOULDER STAND

How Will This Exercise Help?

Tones the entire glandular system by stimulating the thyroid and parathyroid. Improves eyesight, breathing, sexual function, and circulation. Removes fatigue. Improves heart function.

Special Notes

Do not do this exercise if you have neck problems or if you cannot do the Inverted Rest Pose (above). Substitute the Easy Bridge (see p. 118) instead. If you have heart disease or high blood pressure, check with your doctor before trying this exercise. Practice on a soft foam mat or soft carpet to minimize discomfort on the back of your neck.

1. This exercise begins like the Inverted Rest Pose. Sit on the floor with your knees drawn up to your chest and arms wrapped around your knees. Keep your back rounded and your chin tucked into your throat.
2. Gently roll back and forth a few times, rolling onto your upper back and then forward to a sitting position.
3. Now roll back with knees bent and *immediately* support your lower back with your hands (A). Keep your knees bent toward to your forehead at all times.
4. If you feel comfortable, you can *slowly* straighten your legs toward the ceiling and push forward a little on your back with your hands to get as straight as you can comfortably (B). Do not strain! Hold for 15–30 seconds, breathing normally.
5. To come down, fold your knees to your forehead, then gently roll forward into a seated cross-legged position with your head down. Rest for several seconds until your breath returns to normal.

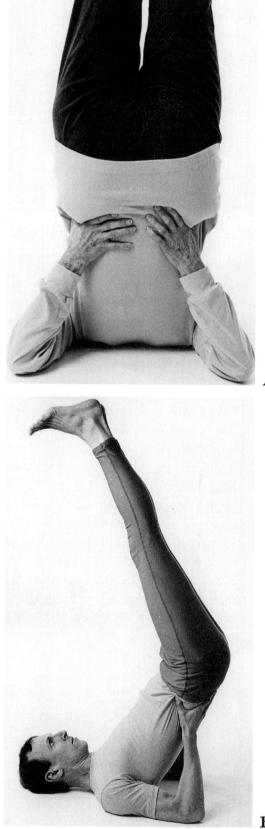

A

B

INCONTINENCE RELIEF

How Will This Exercise Help?

Strengthens all the pelvic and abdominal muscles; if done regularly, can help prevent accidental voiding.

Special Notes

In this exercise, it is important to expel the air completely in Step 3 to achieve the full effect. After tightening your muscles and holding your breath, be sure you release the muscles *before* breathing in. For best results, practice this exercise at least twice a day—more if possible; it can be done conveniently lying in bed just after retiring at night and before getting up in the morning.

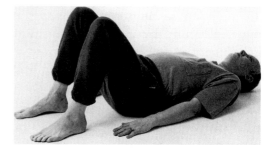

1. Lie flat, with legs bent and feet flat on the bed or floor, separated by several inches. Lay your arms at your sides. Breathe in and out three times through your nose.
2. Breathe out completely, then take a deep breath in through your nose. Hold the breath in for a count of three.
3. Breathe out as hard as you can until all the breath is gone, forcing the breath out until you are completely empty of breath. You will feel your stomach muscles tighten.
4. Holding your breath completely out, suck in all of your stomach, pelvic, and buttock muscles toward your spine as hard as you can. Hold your breath out for a count of three.
5. Release your muscles and breathe in deeply through your nose. Let the breath out normally. Rest a moment, breathing naturally.
6. Repeat for a total of three to five repetitions, resting after each one.

CHAPTER 8

Relaxation and Meditation

"I do my meditation and breathing regularly, and I think my concentration is a lot better, because I'm more aware of things. It's hard to explain, but I noticed it first when driving. It used to be that I never paid much attention to where I was going. But all of a sudden I seem more aware. It's the craziest thing. I notice the street signs and where I'm going. Now I'm taking an interest in things as I never would have before. I think, 'Why am I noticing that? I've gone by here a hundred times, but now it's all new to me!'"

—Doris Manion (age 65)

Taking a few minutes every day to relax and meditate is like taking a refreshing vacation from the stresses and strains of everyday life. One of the most exhausting stresses is the constant mental replay of worries and upsets. Meditation helps you stop the repetition of these irritations in your mind. You will enjoy new, fresh thought and can become aware of the beautiful parts of yourself that you may not have known about before. Regular meditation helps you feel happier about yourself and your life because it teaches you to focus your mental energy on the present rather than worrying about the past or future. If you often experience some of the symptoms of stress, such as rapid heartbeat, "butterflies" in the stomach, tense facial muscles, and so on, try practicing meditation every day and see how easy it becomes to relax your body and mind when you wish. Meditation gives the body and mind a complete rest.

In our American lifestyle, many people do not take the time for daily reflection and silence. We seem to need always to have music playing, or the television or radio on. And yet we spend millions on recreational pursuits such as amusement parks and cruises in our search for ultimate relaxation. Yoga teaches that lasting peace and contentment are found not by going to some place outside yourself but by turning your attention toward inner silence. This takes practice, but most people start feeling benefits the very first time they try it.

If you suffer from chronic pain, insomnia, or other debilitating conditions, you will find relaxation and meditation helpful as well. Relaxation techniques have been applied therapeutically in hospitals and other settings to help alleviate anxiety, pain, hypertension, and other problems. These techniques help you to reduce tension headaches and body aches, to reduce dependence on alcohol, sedatives, or other drugs, and to help yourself deal with many everyday frustrations. Students report that they are less irritable and anxious, and have greater sexual vigor.

There are many misconceptions about meditation, including the belief that it is a religious practice. When religious leaders talk about meditation, they usually use the word to refer to quiet prayer or contemplation with a religious theme. In Yoga, meditation is simply a quieting of one's thoughts, gradually becoming silent, which leads to greater self-awareness, creativity, mental clarity, and intuition. None of my many thousands of students have found any conflict between meditation practice and their chosen faith. Some people believe that meditation is done to music or chanting, but true meditation is never accompanied by music or any other intrusion; you must be quiet and alone for best results.

Meditation develops concentration and alertness. This meditative state is not like sleep; the body completely relaxes, while the mind stays alert but quiet. By creating a quiet, reflective moment in your day, meditation increases your self-understanding. This increased observation of yourself means that you then have the opportunity to develop those parts of yourself that are healthy and enjoyable, such as creativity and helpfulness, and to discard those parts of you that you are not so happy about, such as destructive anger and childish behavior patterns. Meditation allows healing to begin. As you become more aware of your inner self and the depth and beauty inside, you will tend to feel better about yourself. This will reduce feelings of boredom, loneliness, and fear, because you will find that you are happier when you are alone. Meditation improves your intuition, making your hunches more reliable. Most important, meditation practice yields the wisdom to know your true desires and purpose in life. This knowledge allows you to stand proudly and guide the following generations.

In this chapter, you will learn a complete relaxation technique that can be done either lying down on your bed or the floor, or sitting in a chair. Then you will learn two meditation techniques. We have also included some eye exercises in this chapter to help sharpen your concentration.

"My husband died four years ago, and I've been alone since. Last week I had an appointment with a lawyer to make out a will of my own. I was worried that it might be upsetting, so I did my meditation before I went. And you know, it seemed as though my meditation relaxed me enough that the meeting didn't upset me. Any other time I'm sure that type of thing would have bothered me, but it didn't. I really was surprised."

—Pauline Moody (age 73)

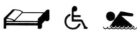

How Will This Exercise Help?

Helps to increase concentration, strengthen the muscles around the eyes, and reduce eyestrain caused by tense muscles. The Eye Palming exercise relieves tension caused by reading, watching television or a computer screen, sewing, or other close work.

Special Notes

These exercises provide a good focusing routine and are best done just prior to relaxation. If you breathe deeply throughout the exercises, this will increase circulation to the eye area and increase the effectiveness of the techniques.

Focusing Exercise

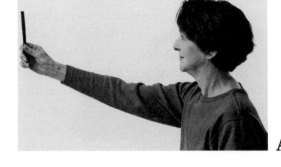

A

1. Hold out a pencil or pen (or even your thumb) at arm's length.
2. Focus your eyes on the tip of the pencil (A).
3. Shift your focus to an object at the far end of the room—for example, a lamp or picture.
4. Shift your focus back and forth from pencil to far wall a few more times. Don't strain.
5. Close your eyes and relax.
6. Breathe in and out deeply several times, then repeat the exercise.

Variation

Focus your eyes on the pencil and slowly move the pencil in toward your nose, keeping your gaze focused on it the whole time. Touch your nose with the pencil. Then move it slowly back out to arm's length. Repeat twice more.

Eye Patterns

1. Sit comfortably straight in your chair. Choose a space such as a door or window frame or a large object such as a television (turned off!).

2. Starting at one corner of the frame, trace the outline of the frame with your eyes, trying to move your eyes very smoothly. Don't strain. Try to move only your eyes, not your entire head.
3. Trace a complete pattern around the object or frame in one direction, then reverse and trace the frame in the opposite direction.
4. Close your eyes and relax. Breathe deeply in and out several times, then repeat the exercise.

Eye Palming

To relieve tension around your eyes at any time of day, place your palms gently over your closed eyes and hold for 10 to 30 seconds (B). Breathe deeply in and out several times.

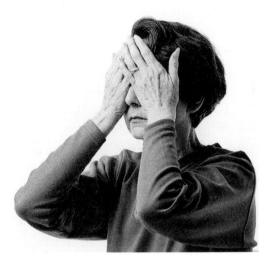

B

"Used to be that after I'd been reading my newspaper for some time the letters would blur—you know, they'd seem to run together until they were just a solid line, no letters left—so I'd have to look off. The Yoga eye exercises are the trick, though. They're real nice. Now if my paper starts to blur I just put it down, sit up, and do those eye rotations up and down, to the sides, you know, about seven, eight times, and then I pick up my paper and start reading again. It seems to strengthen my eyes."

—John Alexander (age 70)

THE COMPLETE RELAXATION PROCEDURE

The ability to relax at will is an important tool among your stress management skills, and this can only be achieved by practicing a little every day. Try to end every exercise session with your complete relaxation technique, followed by 10 to 15 minutes of meditation.

This relaxation technique teaches you how to become aware of muscle tension so you can relax it before it develops into headaches, back pain, or joint stiffness. After you learn the technique, you will be able to use it at other times of the day as well, such as when you feel your muscles becoming tense due to anxiety, or if you have trouble falling asleep or staying asleep. When you are completely relaxed, your body seems to float, or al-

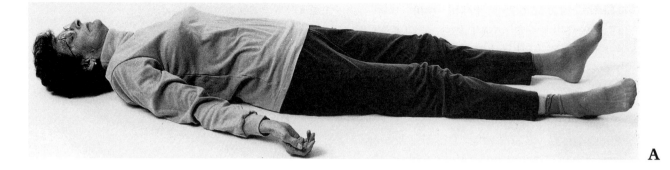

A

most to disappear, and you may forget about it for a few minutes altogether. You may fall asleep for a few moments; this is good for you.

After relaxation, you will go right into meditation practice, so it's important to settle yourself into a comfortable position. Following are some helpful hints for getting the most from your relaxation and meditation practice:

Start in the correct position: You can practice this technique either sitting or lying down. If you lie down on your bed or the floor, lie on your back, and do not use a pillow under your head or neck (A). If your lower back is not comfortable in this position, you may place a pillow under your knees—or use the seated position instead.

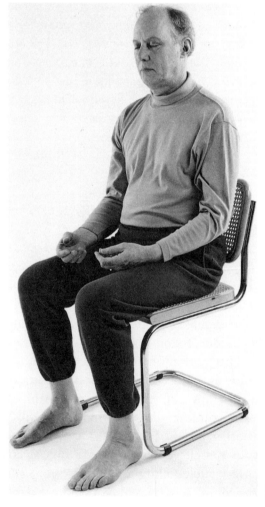

For comfortable posture in a chair, your hips should be pressed against the back of the chair so your spine will remain comfortably straight without slouching or straining (B). Separate your legs a few inches and turn your toes inward so that your knees rest together comfortably. If your back is not comfortable, you may place a small cushion directly behind your lower back, but try to avoid a slouching position.

If you are comfortable getting down on the floor and wish to sit for meditation, sit against a wall with your legs either crossed or extended straight in front of you. Place a pillow behind your lower back for support so your back stays straight.

Stay warm: Wrap up in a sweater or shawl during relaxation and meditation, and wear socks or slippers. When you become very quiet, your body temperature naturally drops slightly, so it is important to stay warm. Also, a wrap provides a psychological feeling of protection while your eyes are closed and you are in a quiet, vulnerable state.

Protect yourself from disturbance: Ask your family to give

B

you these few minutes of quiet time without interruption. Turn off your telephone, and keep pets in another room. Because relaxation and meditation put you into a very quiet state of mind, sudden noises or interruptions can startle you.

Now you are ready to start relaxing. Settle yourself into position, whether seated or lying down, so you are completely comfortable and warm. Take three deep breaths, relaxing more and more with each exhalation.

Read over the following directions and then close your eyes and begin relaxing. In this procedure you will be focusing your attention quietly on each part of your body and visualizing each part in turn. Try to do this without moving any part of your body except your breath. Simply talk to yourself in your mind as you tell yourself to relax each body part. Since you will be doing your relaxation procedure with your eyes closed, read over these instructions several times before you try it. A summary of the relaxation steps appears on p. 138. In the following description, directions for relaxing your physical body are in uppercase type; directions for visualizing your body relaxing are in regular type.

RELAX YOUR FACE FIRST

Gently and calmly bring all of your attention to your forehead. Feel all of the muscles in your forehead. Let them relax so they become loose.

Now become aware of how your eyes feel. Are they tense and jumpy? The eyes are usually the hardest part of the body to relax, so just let them loosen and float in the eye sockets. You aren't going to use your eyes now, so let all tension and movement in the eyes stop. Relax and quiet them. Move on to your lips, teeth, and all the muscles of the jaw, mouth, and throat. Let your tongue relax in your mouth, and say to yourself, "I don't have to speak now for a few minutes." Let all the skin on your face become very loose and still. Let your scalp relax and let your ears droop toward the floor. Your eyes may continue to jump around a little, but don't worry—after some regular practice you will be able to relax them more and more.

RELAX YOUR SHOULDERS, ARMS, AND HANDS

Feel as if you are inside your arms and that they are hollow inside. Let all the muscles of the shoulders settle loosely on the floor. Now move down into your elbow joints and imagine you can see and feel the bones. Let them relax and loosen. Now move down into your forearms, wrists, and right into your hands and fingers, making them hollow, loose, and empty. Relax your fingers completely as though they were empty gloves lying on a table.

RELAX YOUR CHEST

Slowly move your attention into your chest and, for a few moments, just observe the air moving in and out of your lungs like a tiny, warm, relaxing beam of light. Feel your heart beating softly and rhythmically, and notice your belly rising and falling as you breathe. Do not make any attempt to speed up or slow down your breathing. Instead, picture your lungs. Then take in a gentle breath of air, and just as though you are sighing, let the breath out and relax your lungs. Take in another deep, gentle breath, sigh it out, and feel as though your heart also relaxes. Then just let go of your breathing altogether, and relax all tension or effort in your breathing. Observe your belly and try to relax the squeezing effort as you breathe out. Each time you exhale, relax the squeezing of your breath a little more, making it as relaxed as possible so that you are exerting almost no effort or strain to breathe.

RELAX YOUR LEGS

Now, move your attention down into your legs, and make your legs hollow and empty, just as you did with the arms. Loosen and relax your thighs, hip sockets, and groin. Let your legs completely relax and cease moving. Imagine that you are inside your thighs and that they are hollow. Relax your knee joints and feel as though the lower leg is also hollow and empty, all the way into your toes. Imagine your feet are empty with nothing inside, not even any bones. Feel your toenails relax and loosen.

RELAX YOUR SPINE

Now move up your empty feet, legs, and thighs silently, and bring your attention to the base of your spine. Feel your spine and all of its joints from the base of your spine up to the base of your skull at the back of your neck. As you move upward through your waist area, relax any sign of tension so that your entire spine loosens. When you get to the back of your neck, spend a little extra time at this spot. It is a common tension site and needs extra attention. So relax all muscles and tension at the back of your neck where your spine connects to your head. Imagine you can look right down inside of your spinal column as though your spine were a rope dangling down into a dark well. Relax your spine so much that it feels as loose as that rope.

RECHECK YOUR FACE   Now move inside your head, bringing your attention back to your face to see whether or not your face is tense. Relax your eyes even more now, and let them float almost as though you can't feel them move at all.

Before you go on to the next stage, you should quietly observe the entire inside of your body from head to toe. Recheck the three main tension areas: 1) Is your breathing relaxed? 2) Are your eyes and facial muscles relaxed? 3) Is the back of your neck relaxed? Your body will eventually feel as if it were just an empty shell with no tension anywhere. The only movement will be your heart and your breathing, but they also will be very relaxed. Now relax the entire inside of your head. Feel your brain quietly settling inside your head with no effort or strain—just quiet and still.

Here is a summary of the relaxation steps:

1. Relax your face and eyes.
2. Relax and empty your arms and hands.
3. Relax your lungs and heart.
4. Relax your belly and breathing.
5. Relax and empty your legs and feet, especially your thighs and knees.
7. Relax and loosen your back, shoulders, and neck.
8. Relax the inside of your head.
9. Recheck the three major tension areas: (1) your face and eyes; (2) your breathing; (3) the back of your neck.

If you have trouble remembering the sequence of relaxation steps, an easier way to learn is by using a tape. An audiocassette program is available from the American Yoga Association (see Appendix II).

"Several years ago, I was having a great deal of difficulty sleeping. Doctors prescribed drugs, but I still could not get a really restful sleep. I mentioned the problem to my Yoga teacher and she suggested that I meditate myself to sleep. It worked! And the sleep I got was restful. Eight years later, I still use this technique to fall asleep. This technique helped transform what could have been a very debilitating condition into a chance at a new and fuller life."

—Anne Caruso (age 48)

YOUR MEDITATION SESSION

What Is Meditation?

Meditation is simply a quieting of the mind. For about 10 or 15 minutes, try not to think about anything. This is difficult for most people at first, but if you try every day, soon it will become easier and more rewarding.

Start your meditation period by thinking of the sound "Om" (pronounced "ohm"). This word is a sound formula that has a specific effect on the mind when it is repeated or listened to. "Om" is the oldest and most basic sound in classical Yoga. Yogis say that if you could hear the subtle humming sound of the collective atomic structure of your own body and mind, that sound would most resemble the sound "Om."

The "Om" sound of classical Yoga has been adopted and used in a religious way by nearly every religion of the Eastern world to signify one thing or another in their particular theology. However, in classical Yoga, "Om" is used purely as a psychological tool, like a musical note, to center and focus the mind, and is not meant to indicate any particular religious concept or deity. Its purpose is simply to empty the mind except for the sound itself.

The purely psychological aspects of "Om" were described more than 2,500 years ago in the Manduka Upanishad, where "Om" is interpreted allegorically to possess four distinct elements pertaining to four different states of consciousness. The first part of "Om," the "A" sound, is said to signify our conscious self when we are awake. The second part, the "U" sound, is said to signify our subconscious self, when we are asleep and dreaming. The third aspect of "Om," the "M" sound, is said to signify our unconscious self, when we are in deep dreamless sleep. The fourth aspect of "Om," represented by the silence before and after the word, is said to signify that portion of ourselves that exists in absolute silence of mind in what is called our witness consciousness. Hence, by the repetition and focusing upon "Om," one's mind is led gently into a timeless peace and silence, which leads to greater knowledge of our own self.

When you practice meditation, you will probably find that your experience of silence will be deeper and more refreshing if you repeat "Om" to yourself several times at the beginning of your meditation session. Then simply stop talking to yourself in your mind. Try to stop all inner conversation. Don't force it; you will probably be quiet for a few seconds, then a thought will come into your mind; it may be several more seconds before you realize that you are thinking again. When you do notice that you are thinking, just let the thought trail away in your mind, and go back to the idea of silence. This will happen several times during your meditation period. Don't worry about this; meditation is a process, not a forced goal to add stress to your life! Treat your daily meditation session as a game; see how long you can be still before a thought interrupts you. Some days you will be able to be still for a long time; other days it will seem as if you can't stop thinking even for a second. Just keep trying every day and focus on the refreshing, quiet feeling that stays with you after your meditation session. Eventually you will notice that this feeling can accompany you throughout your day. All you have to do is remember the feeling, and it will be there. Many students tell me that their daily meditation period is as refreshing as a short nap! It is a tremendous help to concentration.

Don't worry if you fall asleep during meditation at first. This is natural, because your body is receiving all the normal signals of sleep: eyes closed, body relaxed, and so forth. Just keep meditating, and eventually your body will learn to rest deeply while your mind remains alert and focused on silence.

Decide before you start meditation how long you are going to remain quiet. It is not a good idea to use a clock or timer, because the loud noise will startle you. The best way is to tell yourself before you begin how long you wish to meditate. Then your mind will automatically come out of meditation at that time.

For best results, try to meditate for at least 10 minutes at first. Later, when the process becomes more comfortable, you can extend your meditation period to 20 or 30 minutes, or even longer if you wish.

"I use the meditation to help control my asthma. Most of my asthma problems, and most of my problems in general, are caused by nerves and depression, and I've noticed a big improvement in that area. The biggest thing anybody can do is to relax, so the meditation really helps me."
—Alice Blauvelt (age 66)

AFTER MEDITATION

The way you come out of meditation is as important as the way you relax into it. If you get up too quickly, or disturb yourself too abruptly, you may become jittery or upset. Before you start to move around, lie still for a few minutes longer thinking about the sensations, emotional feelings, and thoughts that you experienced during your meditation period. Don't just jump up out of meditation. Increase your breathing first, and that will start to reactivate everything else. At first, when you go to move your hands and arms, they may feel a little like wood since they've become so utterly relaxed. Stretch your arms and legs as a cat does when it awakens from a nap. Give yourself time to reenter your normal activities refreshed, alert, and recharged with new energy and a clear mind.

THE "I LOVE YOU" FANTASY TECHNIQUE

The "I Love You" fantasy technique, practiced regularly, will help to reinforce feelings of self-confidence, raise self-esteem, remove fear, and reduce the incidence of crippling "ugly fits." This technique should be done as a complement to—rather than as a substitute for—your daily meditation period.

Start with the Laughing Bicycle (for illustration, see p. 83): Lying on your back (or seated in a chair), pump your legs as if you were riding a bicycle. Pump your arms as well, and laugh out loud for several seconds. Then relax and settle into a comfortable position. This exercise helps to release tension and stimulates the brain chemicals that cause feelings of well-being.

Give yourself the same protections as when you are doing your regular meditation: Lie on your back comfortably, without a pillow under your head, on your bed or the floor, or sit in a chair that keeps your back straight. Cover yourself with a blanket or shawl. Make sure your pets are in another room and turn off your telephone.

Press your back slightly toward the floor (or the back of the chair), then release and relax. Pull your chin down a little toward your chest without straining, to stretch the cords in the back of the neck that will allow more movement of the feeling that is going to affect your brain. If you are lying down and your lower back is tense, place one or two pillows under your knees.

Read through the instructions a few times so that you can go through the exercise with your eyes closed. The directions follow somewhat the same pattern as the Complete Relaxation Procedure: You start with your face, continue down to your feet, and move back up your spine to your head again. In this exercise, however, you use your breath and the words "I love you" to relax each part of your body. If you have trouble remembering the sequence of steps, an audiocassette program is available from the American Yoga Association (see Appendix II).

| BEGIN BY BRINGING YOUR ATTENTION TO YOUR FOREHEAD | Breathe in, saying "I love you" to yourself as you breathe in. Then say "I love you" as you breathe out. Repeat several times. Now breathe in and hold for a moment. Imagine the feeling "I |

love you" spreading throughout your brain as a beautiful, warm, wet, perfumed essence. Breathe out "I love you."

NOW RELAX COMPLETELY. LET YOUR BREATH RELAX

And just hold that feeling. For a few more minutes, continue saying "I love you" as you breathe in and out.

Now think to yourself as you breathe in and hold your breath for a moment: "Whom do I love?" Breathe out and say "I love you." Breathe in and hold again; think: "Who loves me?" Now think to yourself: "My breath loves me." Breathe out. "My breath loves me." The breath is inside you. It loves you. Breathe in and think "I'm holding my breath—it loves me." Breathe out and think "I have released my breath—it still loves me." Take a deep breath, always through your nose. Breathe in: "My breath loves me." Breathe out: "My breath is gone now and it still loves me."

NOW RELAX COMPLETELY. VISUALIZE THE INSIDE OF YOUR HEAD AND YOUR BODY

Think of how the breath is commingled with love. Oxygen is flowing through your veins and heart and every part of you because you can't live without your breath. Visualize this loving breath inside your body. Are there any impediments keeping it from moving where it wants to go? Visualize this feeling of love and breath removing any kind of block or constriction, moving easily and sweetly throughout your body.

BRING THE BREATH TO YOUR FOREHEAD

Think "I love you—my breath is in my forehead." Relax your forehead. Think of this feeling of love spreading to your eyes—you can almost see it!

RELAX YOUR EYES	Let the breath of love flow out into the rest of your face. Feel it in your nose, because it breathes for you. Every time you breathe in, breathe "I love you." Every time you breathe out, breathe "I love you." Let the breath of love flow freely so that your face melts with love.
LET YOUR MOUTH AND THROAT RELAX	Think "I love you" as you breathe.
LET YOUR NECK RELAX NOW	Relax so that no constriction can stop the breath from moving. Love comes in with your breath—relax. Love goes out with your breath—relax.
RELAX YOUR COLLARBONE	Relax it toward the floor and say "I love you." Let the ends of your shoulders relax.
RELAX YOUR ARMS	Feel that they are fully supported by this breath of love. Rest your arms in love.
RELAX YOUR WRISTS	Let your hands be totally relaxed in love. You're vulnerable. You don't care. You can't lose love. Breath comes in and it goes out, and love is still there.
RELAX YOUR FINGERS	Let them curl slightly, like a baby's hands.
BRING YOUR ATTENTION TO YOUR CHEST	Be aware that you are taking a breath into your heart: "I love you." Breathe it out with love. Breathe into your lungs: "I love you." Breathe out: "I love you." Now relax your entire chest. Let your breath relax in love. Become aware that this breath is love. You're not making it happen; it's happening because it loves you.
BREATHE IN AND THINK OF YOUR STOMACH	Breathe out and say "I love you" as you relax your stomach. Relax your abdomen, thinking: "I love you. I love you the way you are." Now feel the breath of love move through your hip

	joints. Warm, liquid, beautiful—perfectly balanced and poised.
RELAX YOUR HIPS	Now say "I love you" to your hips and let the large bones in the top of your legs sink toward the floor; you don't have to hold them up. You love them. They love you. You can't lose love.
RELAX YOUR LEGS	Relax them in love.
RELAX YOUR KNEES AND ANKLES	Relax them and think "I love you."
RELAX YOUR FEET	Now think to your feet "I love you."
BRING YOUR ATTENTION UP TO THE BACK OF YOUR HIPS AND THE BASE OF YOUR SPINE	Now picture yourself just simply floating; completely supported on this breath, this love. Open up this hip/spine area like a flower. Say "I love you." Don't fight it. Let it flow easily, smooth and quiet.
RELAX THE BACK OF YOUR SHOULDER BLADES	Let your back become soft. Love is supporting you. "I love you, back."
THE BACK OF YOUR NECK RELAXES	Think to yourself, "I love you. I love you." Then reach your brain, your hair, all soft and supported, resting in love, in breath.

Breathe in and think love. Breathe out—love is still there. Think of your brain floating in a pool of this love. Now make it totally quiet and say to yourself, "I love you." Bring your mind to your forehead and think nothing. Hold this feeling. If you feel any other thought coming in, make sure that it says "I love you." Transpose any thought to "I love you" and go back to thinking nothing. Think nothing for as long as you can. Stop talking to yourself. Become silent internally.

Rest quietly like this for about 10 minutes, then slowly stretch, take a deep breath and let it out, and think about how you feel. Rest on your side or stomach for a few minutes, enjoying the feeling before you get up. Move slowly back into your normal attitudes and lifestyle.

"It clears up my thinking. I just shut my eyes and relax, and it stops everything from moving so fast, it really does. I just feel that there's more

joy in me, it's so peaceful, and that relaxed feeling that I had while I was practicing comes over me later and helps me keep going. And because of that I can express myself better than before. It's as though it was crowded inside me—now it's more open and I have happier communications with people."

—Gene Roy (age 62)

CHAPTER 9

Diet and Nutrition

"The doctor said Harry's blood sugar was too high, so we decided that we'd go without sugar. We made a study of it by reading the labels. You'd be surprised how many things have sugar in them, and a lot of it! One thing I watch most of all is the cereal. We could only find two that don't contain sugar. I make sure that nothing we eat has sugar in it. And do you know what's happened? Harry's blood sugar level went right back down where it should be, and we lost weight fast! We didn't intend to lose weight, we just did it for our health. It is surely the easiest way to lose weight that there is!"

—Harry and Clara Harvey, Alice Christensen's parents
(ages 84 and 82)

Most people know they should improve their diet, but most people also believe that to do so they must give up their favorite foods and resign themselves to tasteless, unappetizing meals.

Not so! Eating healthier foods does not have to be a hardship. It will pay off in weight loss, more energy, less illness, and a generally more youthful feeling. In this chapter you will find some simple suggestions for gradually making some changes in how you choose, prepare, and eat foods, and some new ways to look at what food does for you, both physically and mentally.

It just makes sense that if you are trying to improve your health by practicing Yoga exercise, breathing, and meditation, you also want to feed your body foods that will do the same thing. Combining good nutrition with a safe, gentle exercise program means that you are doubling your efforts toward good health, enhancing the feeling that you are taking care of yourself.

Exercise alone can improve muscle tone and strength, and well-conditioned muscles burn more calories, improve posture, and give you a more fit appearance. Your food choices can help or hinder this process. For instance, all women begin to lose bone density at around age thirty. The problem can develop into osteoporosis (brittle bones) in later life if it is not addressed early on. It takes a combination of weight-bearing exercise and added calcium in the diet to prevent this common problem.

The constantly evolving science of nutrition has uncovered a direct relationship between malnutrition and illness. The illnesses caused by malnutrition shorten life and make existence painful and unhappy. In addition to hampering efforts at weight management, eating too much fat, calories, salt, sugar, and cholesterol can contribute to diseases such as cancer, stroke, heart disease, high blood pressure, and diabetes. Similarly, a diet that is low in protein, iron, and vitamins A, B complex, and C can contribute to problems such as anemia, excessive fatigue, depression, and poor resistance to infection. Simply increasing dietary fiber and drinking more water (along with regular exercise) can often alleviate constipation.

Here are concrete suggestions to help us live longer and better:

- Do not abuse alcohol or drugs.
- Avoid tobacco completely.
- Avoid being overweight and following fad diets.
- Eat a low-fat diet consisting primarily of fresh fruits and vegetables, whole-grain products, eggs, and low-fat dairy products.
- Take a balanced vitamin/mineral supplement daily and a separate tablet or powder with extra vitamin C.
- Before age forty-five, eat a high-protein diet; after forty-five, eat a lower-protein diet.
- Exercise daily.
- Get adequate rest and relaxation.
- Seek and follow qualified medical treatment, and beware of medical quackery.

SIMPLE GUIDELINES FOR EATING BETTER

Drink less caffeine (coffee, tea, colas); instead, drink skim milk, fruit juices, or flavored but unsugared sparkling water. Drink more plain water, too. New studies show that older adults don't get as thirsty as younger people, so they may not drink enough to prevent dehydration. A good rule of thumb is to drink more than what you feel you need to quench your thirst, especially during and after exercising.

Eat less meat (especially high-fat, processed varieties such as bacon, hot dogs, sausage, fatback, cold cuts); instead, eat low-fat or nonfat dairy foods, nutritional yeast (p. 153), and soy products such as tofu (p. 152).

Eat less canned or prepared fruits and vegetables; instead, buy fresh produce (provided you can eat it within a few days) and frozen fruits and vegetables if you shop less frequently.

Eat less white bread and high-fat bakery items such as muffins and croissants, and eat less white rice, white pasta, and refined cereals; instead, make or buy whole-grain breads, muffins, cereals, and pancakes, and eat brown or wild rice and whole-grain pasta. Head for the health food section!

Avoid lard or other meat fat, and cut down on butter, margarine (both have the same calories), and shortening (these "hydrogenated" fats are also found in most packaged snack foods and bakery goods). Substitute small amounts of vegetable oils that contain less saturated fat, such as olive, canola, sunflower, safflower, peanut, sesame, or walnut oil. (All oils have the same number of calories, but those with highest saturated fat are the most likely to contribute to heart disease and other problems.) Don't be tempted by the new fat substitutes such as Olestra. Their effects have not been adequately tested, and many people report digestive problems with their use. Also, some studies have shown that Olestra removes some of the essential fat-soluble vitamins (A, D, and E) from the body. When sautéing or greasing a pan, use a vegetable oil spray.

Note: If you are underweight, or if you have recently lost weight due to illness, include a moderate amount of fat in your diet to help you regain a normal weight. The best way to gain weight is to eat an extra snack each day and add a little extra food to each meal. Don't skip meals. Try to add high-carbohydrate foods, such as fruits and starchy vegetables along with whole-grain foods like bread, pancakes, and cereal, to get the extra calories you need.

Cut down on sugar and sweet, high-fat desserts; instead, substitute fresh fruit, or make your own desserts: You can easily cut the added sweeteners up to half the amount called for in the recipe, and use plain, nonfat yogurt or apple butter instead of butter or oil. Slightly increase vanilla and sweet spices such as cinnamon to enhance the sweet taste. Be careful of artificial sweeteners; some contain cancer-causing chemicals.

Cut down on sodium by reducing your consumption of salty snacks, processed foods, and fast food.

Eat less at night when you're inactive. Follow the old saying: "Eat breakfast like a king, lunch like a prince, and supper like a pauper." If you have the willpower to eat six small, nutritious meals instead of three big ones, without adding calories, that's even healthier. A great evening snack is a big tray of fresh vegetables with a low-fat dip made with cottage cheese and any seasonings you like.

Avoid artificial "chemical" foods and overprocessed foods (margarine, nondairy creamers, nondairy dessert toppings, imitation juices, diet soft drinks, and artificially colored and flavored foods). Artificial color and flavor cause allergic reactions in some people.

Eat more fiber and protein to prevent constipation and protect against cancer and heart disease. Some high-fiber foods (starting with those having the highest content) are 100 percent bran cereal, kidney and lima beans, lentils, barley, almonds, corn, peas, apples, prunes, Shredded Wheat, oranges, peaches, potatoes (with skin), bananas, and broccoli. The recommended daily intake of fiber is about 20–30 grams—about twice what most people eat on average. To increase your fiber intake, every day eat a high-fiber cereal, 2 servings of whole-grain bread or rolls, 2 servings of fruit (not juice), and 3 servings of vegetables (such as salad, hearty soup, and raw or cooked vegetables).

Eat more beans and peas. Use canned or frozen varieties to save soaking and cooking time (drain and rinse thoroughly to reduce gas). Use in salads, soups, casseroles, or puree with lemon and spices in a food processor to make a dip for fresh vegetables.

SOME FACTS ABOUT SUGAR

- "Raw" sugar isn't raw—it's just partly refined, and no better for you than white sugar. Brown sugar is just white sugar coated with molasses. Honey contains some trace nutrients and tastes sweeter than sugar, so you may use less of it. Blackstrap molasses contains iron, calcium, and potassium.
- Sugar-coated cereal contains about 5 teaspoons of sugar per cup.
- A 12-ounce can of cola contains about 10 teaspoons of sugar.
- Try not to get hooked on artificial sweeteners; saccharin (Sweet'n Low) is potentially cancer-causing, and NutraSweet (Equal) is suspected of causing headaches and other side effects in some people.
- If you are constantly craving sugar, your diet is probably inadequate, especially in the B-complex vitamins and protein. Read the books suggested at the end of this chapter, or ask a competent nutritionist to make a plan for you.

HOW MUCH OF EACH FOOD?

In the previous section I suggested that you eat more of this and less of that—but how much should you eat? It can be confusing when you try to plan a balanced diet with so many variables. The food guide pyramid promoted by the U.S. Department of Agriculture and modified by various medical and nutrition organizations helps to organize the number of servings of different kinds of food to include in your diet every day.

The largest section of the pyramid is the category of bread, cereal, pasta, and baked goods, and the recommendation is to eat 6 to 11 servings every day. One serving consists of:

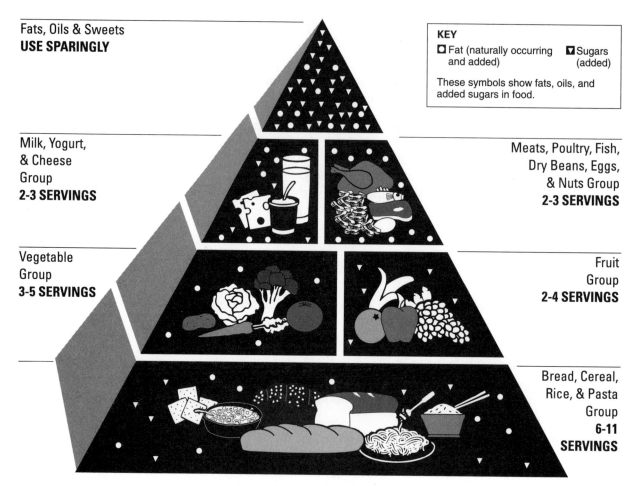

Fats, Oils & Sweets
USE SPARINGLY

Milk, Yogurt,
& Cheese
Group
2-3 SERVINGS

Meats, Poultry, Fish,
Dry Beans, Eggs,
& Nuts Group
2-3 SERVINGS

Vegetable
Group
3-5 SERVINGS

Fruit
Group
2-4 SERVINGS

Bread, Cereal,
Rice, & Pasta
Group
**6-11
SERVINGS**

Source: U.S. Department of Agriculture &
U.S. Department of Health and Human Services

> 1 slice bread
> 1/2 cup rice or pasta (cooked)
> 1 ounce cereal (1/4 to 2 cups, depending on brand)
> 1/2 bagel or muffin
> 1 small tortilla
> 5 crackers
> small handful pretzels

You can see that a normal portion of rice or pasta is more like 1 or 1 1/2 cups, so you get more than one serving out of that meal. A day's menu that included cereal for breakfast, a sandwich for lunch, crackers for a snack, and spaghetti for dinner would count as 6 servings of grains.

The next category on the food pyramid is vegetables, and the recommended daily number of servings is 3 to 5. A serving consists of:

> 1 cup raw leafy vegetables (such as salad)
> 1/2 cup chopped raw or cooked vegetables
> 1 medium carrot

1 large celery stalk

$^1/_2$ acorn squash

6 ounces vegetable juice

This portion of your daily diet would be satisfied by eating tomato and lettuce slices on your sandwich, a cup of tomato juice for a snack, and a salad and a cooked vegetable at dinner. I would encourage you to eat as much as you want in this category.

Fruits are the next category, with the recommendation that we eat 2 to 4 servings per day. One serving consists of:

1 medium whole fruit

$^1/_2$ cup cooked fruit

wedge of melon

$^3/_4$ cup fruit juice

$^1/_4$ cup dried fruit such as raisins, prunes, and so on

Add a glass of juice at breakfast and fruit for dessert at lunch, and you've had 2 servings of fruit for the day. Fresh fruits and vegetables should not be washed until just before using. Store them in the refrigerator or other cold, dark place, and use within a few days to retain as many of the nutrients as possible. Serve them raw, washed in cold running water; or cook them by rapid steaming (inexpensive vegetable steamers are available from most stores). This waterless method preserves the flavor, color, and nutritional content of your food. If possible, do not peel vegetables, or, instead, peel them after cooking, just before serving.

The next group is dairy foods. Your recommended 2 to 3 servings of dairy foods can be fulfilled by adding milk to your cereal, a slice of cheese to your sandwich, and a sprinkling of Parmesan cheese to your spaghetti. This is an easy category to eat too much of, so concentrate on low-fat or nonfat dairy products.

The next group encompasses meat, poultry, fish, dried beans, eggs, and nuts, and the recommendation is to eat 2 to 3 servings per day. You don't need to rely on meat for your main source of protein. You can easily fulfill this dietary requirement by including a veggie burger or veggie dog on your lunch sandwich and 2 tablespoons of peanut butter on your snack crackers. Add $^1/_2$ cup of lentil soup, and you've easily met your daily goal.

At the very top of the pyramid are fats, oils, and sweets, to be eaten sparingly, especially if you are trying to lose weight. Try a low-fat dressing on your salad, or make your own dressing with a little olive oil and an interesting vinegar. See the suggestions elsewhere in this chapter for modifying dessert recipes (p. 148) and trying different toppings for baked potatoes (p. 155).

If you add up the servings described above, your menu for the day looks like this:

Breakfast: High-fiber cereal with sliced peaches and nonfat milk; glass of orange juice.

Snack: Whole-grain crackers with a small amount of old-fashioned peanut butter (with no added fat); glass of tomato juice.

Lunch: Veggie burger on whole-grain bun topped with lettuce and tomato slices and a slice of cheese; cup of lentil soup; glass of nonfat milk.

Dinner: Spaghetti with tomato sauce and broccoli florets; mixed green salad with low-calorie dressing; fresh strawberries.

SUPER FOODS

Some foods are so loaded with nutrients that you should try to eat them every day. They are:

- *Milk.* A quart of milk contains all the vitamin D you need for the day, plus about two-thirds of your protein and calcium requirements. Milk also contains several important B vitamins and potassium. Many people don't drink milk because they believe it causes gas and bloating. Usually this is not a problem if you drink one glass at a time. There are also lactose-free brands of milk or over-the-counter additives to help with digestion; yogurt or buttermilk are also good substitutes. Choose skim or 1 percent milk.

- *Greens.* Collards, spinach, and kale are excellent sources of folic acid, vitamin C, potassium, and beta-carotene. Collards and kale also provide calcium. Lutein, a substance found in greens, may reduce the risk of macular degeneration, a common cause of blindness in older adults. Many nutrition experts believe that foods in the cabbage family, including collard greens and kale along with broccoli, cauliflower, and brussels sprouts, help protect us from cancer.

- *Whole-grain or high-fiber breakfast cereals.* Most of these are fortified with vitamin D, folic acid, and several other vitamins and minerals. Also, they can help prevent constipation.

- *Soy products* such as tofu and soy powder are cheap, low-fat sources of protein. They can be a good source of calcium if processed with calcium sulfate (check the label). Add soy powder (found in health food stores) to baked goods such as muffins and breads. It can also be added to blender drinks such as yogurt smoothies. Tofu comes in block or crumbled form. It is tasteless until cooked with seasonings such as onions, garlic, and spices. It is excellent steamed or lightly sautéed and combined with vegetables and rice or pasta, or use it as a substitute for meat in chili, soups and stews, and casseroles. Lightly sauté strips of tofu in a little olive oil with seasonings, drain between paper towels, and use in sandwiches instead of lunch meats or high-fat cheese.

- *Nutritional yeast.* This is not the same as baking yeast. Nutritional yeast is specially grown for nutritional purposes and is found in powder or flake form (tablets are also available, but they are not as effective). The best source of all the B-complex vitamin team, nutritional yeast is also a very good, low-fat source of protein. Add it to your diet slowly, starting with one teaspoonful mixed in unsweetened fruit juice or water before a meal, like a cocktail. Slowly increase this amount to 1 tablespoon, three times a day. Ask your health food store or pharmacy to order primary-type brewer's yeast. There are many brands on the market. Buy small quantities until you find the one you like best. Our favorite brand is NBC 600 Red Star from Walnut Acres, a mail-order natural foods company in Penns Creek, PA.

MENUS AND PREPARATION TIPS

Here are some additional suggestions for varying your meals without sacrificing taste or nutrients. I recommend that you begin every meal with at least 1 teaspoon of nutritional yeast stirred into a glass of fruit juice or water.

Breakfast Menu Suggestions

A teaspoon or two of wheat germ, an excellent source of iron, vitamin E, and B-complex vitamins, can be added to pancake mixes or sprinkled on cottage cheese, yogurt, or cereal. Begin every day with a nutritional yeast "cocktail." To make this, in a blender or a glass mix together 1 or 2 teaspoons of nutritional yeast with fruit juice, water, or milk. Gradually increase the amount to 1 tablespoon.

1.
Cottage cheese or yogurt with fresh fruit
Whole-wheat toast with one teaspoon of butter or fruit-
   only preserves
2.
Unsweetened fruit juice
Oatmeal or other whole-grain cereal such as Ralston or
   Wheatena, cooked with skim milk instead of water, and
   flavored with fruit, a little dark brown sugar or honey, and
   raisins, nuts, or sunflower seeds

3.

Soft-boiled, poached, or scrambled eggs (limit: 4–6 eggs
    weekly)

Whole-grain bagel or toast with fruit-only preserves

4.

Whole-grain or buckwheat pancakes or waffles topped with
    stewed fruit such as applesauce

Glass of buttermilk or skim milk, or serving of cottage
    cheese

5.

1 ounce hard cheese and tomato slices broiled on whole-
    wheat toast

Fruit smoothie: in blender, whirl fresh fruit, yogurt or skim
    milk, cracked ice, and a teaspoon of honey, if desired, until
    smooth (or use frozen fruit and omit ice)

6.

Whole-grain cold cereal without added sugar such as
    Grape-Nuts, Shredded Wheat, or All-Bran, served with
    skim milk, sliced banana, and raisins (avoid granolas,
    because they usually have a very high sugar and fat
    content)

Lunch Menu Suggestions

Instead of soft drinks, have skim milk, buttermilk, fruit or vegetable juices, or sparkling water flavored with lemon. If you drink
coffee or tea, make it decaffeinated.

1.

Open-faced sandwich topped with lots of vegetables such as
    mushrooms, onions, tomatoes, and peppers, topped with 1
    ounce cheese and broiled

Fresh fruit salad

2.

Big, fresh, green salad with 1 ounce low-fat grated cheese,
    vegetables, a few olives, 1 tablespoon homemade or low-
    fat oil-and-vinegar dressing

Bran muffin

3.

Hearty vegetable soup made with brown rice and red
    kidney beans

Whole-wheat crackers and 1 ounce cheese

4.

Noodle or rice casserole (whole-wheat noodles or brown
    rice are best) including vegetables such as peas, green

peppers, mushrooms, broccoli, or cauliflower, a small
amount of cheese, and sauce made from low-fat canned
cream soup (can be made ahead of time, frozen in small
servings, and reheated in the microwave or toaster oven)

5.

A steamed vegetable such as broccoli, cauliflower, brussels
sprouts, or greens, broiled with a little olive oil, lemon
juice, seasonings, and a sprinkling of bread crumbs
Sliced fresh tomatoes topped with cottage cheese
Whole-wheat roll

6.

Baked potato topped with plenty of seasonings and one or
more of the following: vegetable stew or chili; low-fat
cheese; steamed vegetables such as broccoli; low-fat
yogurt, low-fat sour cream, or cottage cheese; a drizzle of
olive oil; lemon juice
Fresh fruit salad

Dinner Menu Suggestions

Cook one package (2 cups) of brown rice every week and keep it
in a tightly closed container in the refrigerator. Use it with vegetable stew, boiled beans, greens, and soups throughout the week
to add fiber and flavor to your meals. If you prefer a small glass of
wine with dinner, drink an extra glass of water also.

1.

Succotash made with lima beans, whole-kernel corn, and
red pimentos
Whole-grain rolls
Fresh coleslaw with low-fat dressing
Fresh fruit salad with yogurt dressing

2.

Mixed vegetable soup or low-fat creamed soup
Broiled cheese and tomato open-faced sandwich

3.

Three-bean salad made with low-fat Italian dressing
Cheese toast
Fresh fruit

4.

Broiled mustard or turnip greens sautéed in a little olive oil
with onions, garlic, and spices, and seasoned with vinegar
or lemon juice
Cottage cheese
Corn bread

5.

Spinach salad with whole-grain croutons, tomatoes,
   avocados, and onions, topped with low-calorie mustard
   dressing
Cottage cheese and fresh fruit

Snack Suggestions

Glass of buttermilk or skim milk or nutritional yeast drink, plus
one of the following:

- Handful of roasted soy beans, sunflower seeds, and nuts
- Peanut butter (use an old-fashioned brand without added fat)
  on whole-wheat bread, whole-wheat crackers, or celery
- All you want of raw carrots, celery, and other vegetables and
  fresh fruits

NUTRITION GLOSSARY

Here are descriptions of some essential nutrients and suggestions
for obtaining them from the foods you eat. Since it is almost im-
possible to eat everything you need every day for a perfectly balanced diet, health professionals often recommend supplementing
the diet with a good multivitamin and mineral tablet. Look for
brands that include the following recommended amounts of essential nutrients:

vitamin A (beta-carotene) 5000 IU
vitamins B_1, B_2, B_6 (10 mg each)
vitamin B_3 (50 mg)
vitamin B_{12} (25 mcg)
biotin (200 mcg)
pantothenic acid (50 mcg)
folic acid (400 mcg)
vitamin C (500 mg)
vitamin E (200–400 IU)
vitamin D (400 IU)
calcium (800 mg)
magnesium (300 mg; about one-half the amount of calcium)

Note: Few multivitamins have enough vitamin E, C, calcium, or
magnesium; you may have to take them separately. Since you
probably get plenty of iron in your food, look for a supplement
that contains little or no iron.

Remember that a daily vitamin/mineral tablet is no substitute
for a balanced diet, since food contains many helpful substances

that have not yet been isolated. Use your daily vitamin/mineral supplement as a type of insurance that you are getting adequate amounts of the most important nutrients.

Vitamin A prevents infections, maintains acute vision, and keeps the skin beautiful. Foods rich in vitamin A are eggs, cheese, and butter; some margarines and milk are fortified with vitamin A. Orange, yellow, and dark green fruits and vegetables are rich in beta-carotene (which converts to vitamin A in your body). Beta-carotene in supplement form does not appear to be toxic, but vitamin A (from palmitate or fish-liver oils) can be toxic if taken in large doses for an extended time.

Vitamin B complex is important for healthy nerves, proper digestion, and energy. Foods rich in B-complex vitamins are fortified cereals, nutritional yeast, whole grains, nuts, and seeds. Yogurt, buttermilk, and cottage cheese establish bacteria in your intestines that produce B vitamins. Vitamin B_{12} is especially important for older adults, whose bodies often don't absorb enough from food. Memory loss and confusion are some symptoms of early B_{12} deficiency. Be sure your vitamin/mineral tablet includes 15–25 micrograms (mcg) of B_{12}.

Because the B vitamins are water soluble, they pass through the system quickly. People who are inactive do not have the same fluid movement through the body, and so they do not absorb nutrients as efficiently as younger people. For these reasons, it would be better to take a low-potency tablet three or more times per day than it would be to take a high-potency tablet once per day.

Folic Acid, a B vitamin, is a nutrient that helps prevent heart disease and stroke. It can also help with difficulties in digestion such as diarrhea. Folate-rich foods include (in decreasing order) fortified cereals, nutritional yeast, lentils and other legumes, spinach and other greens, orange juice, peas, and other vegetables. Your vitamin/mineral supplement should provide you with the USRDA of 400 mcg.

Vitamin C repairs bones, cartilage, spinal disks, and blood vessels. It breaks up blood fats, increases the antiarthritic hormones, and helps fight harmful bacteria and viruses. Foods rich in vitamin C are fruits and vegetables, especially citrus fruits and greens. If you decide to supplement your diet, choose quick-dissolving tablets of plain ascorbic acid (the cheapest brands are fine; no need to spend extra money on extra ingredients) or crystals that can be mixed into water or juice.

Calcium and magnesium are natural tranquilizers, and they keep the bones and teeth strong. Calcium-rich food sources are dairy foods; dark green, leafy vegetables; nuts; tofu (processed with calcium sulphate); and whole grains. Most people, especially older adults, do not get enough calcium in their diets. The RDA for older adults is 800 mg. When shopping for an extra calcium supplement, choose calcium from milk (lactate) or oyster shell (oxalate) sources rather than dolomite, which may contain lead; the product should also contain about half as much magnesium as calcium.

Chromium is necessary for metabolism of carbohydrates. Foods rich in chromium are nutritional yeast, cheese, dried beans, peanuts, and whole-grain breads and cereals. A good multivitamin/mineral supplement includes the USRDA of 50–200 mcg of chromium.

Vitamin D is needed to absorb calcium, which increases bone density. Foods rich in vitamin D are fortified milk and cereals. Under certain conditions it is produced on the skin by sunshine. Vitamin D is toxic if taken as a supplement at high doses for extended periods. Older adults do not generally absorb vitamin D from food as well as younger people, so they are more likely to be deficient. If you are taking a multivitamin supplement, it probably contains the USRDA of 400 IU of vitamin D.

Vitamin E is an antioxidant that helps boost the immune system, prevents scarring, prevents muscle damage from vigorous exercise, and protects various nutrients and hormones from being destroyed by oxygen. It also reduces muscle cramps and restless legs. Foods rich in vitamin E are whole-grain cereals and breads, dried beans, green leafy vegetables, and wheat germ. It has been suggested that, because our immune systems become less efficient as we age, we should probably supplement our diet with extra vitamin E. Most vitamin/mineral supplements include the USRDA of 30 IU of vitamin E, but many authorities recommend that seniors take between 200 and 400 IU for extra protection.

Fluoride helps to form strong bones and teeth. Drinking fluoridated water (most municipalities add fluoride to their water systems) will provide you with an adequate amount. Bottled waters do not contain fluoride.

Iodine increases your energy and boosts circulation. Iodized salt will supply you with adequate iodine.

Iron prevents a type of anemia that can be recognized by pallor, shortness of breath, brittle nails, heart palpitations, forgetfulness, and depression. Foods rich in iron are blackstrap molasses, nutritional yeast, wheat germ, and wheat bran. Most breakfast cereals are fortified with iron. About 4 to 6 percent of women and 2 percent of men are iron-deficient, but check with your doctor before supplementing; since the greatest concentrations of iron are found in beef, bread and rolls, fortified cereals, and crackers, most people get quite enough in their diet. Most babies who are called "colicky" and can't sleep suffer from iron deficiency.

Lecithin, often extracted from soybeans, is an emulsifier of blood fats. It helps prevent the cholesterol deposits that cause hardening of the arteries. The B vitamins in lecithin also help protect the liver from cirrhosis. Granular lecithin can be obtained from your pharmacy or health food store; it also can be taken in capsule form. Keep it refrigerated. The granular form can be added to blender drinks, sprinkled on cereal or in soups, or just stirred into your nutritional yeast cocktail.

Protein is necessary for maintaining muscle mass and a healthy immune system, and protecting against stress. Most people can get enough protein from their diet unless they are eating too little food altogether, but older adults who are frail or whose incomes are low are more at risk of not getting enough protein. The trick is to get adequate protein without the extra fat that accompanies the highest sources of protein—namely, meat and high-fat cheeses. Some good, low-fat, inexpensive sources of protein are low-fat or nonfat dairy foods, legumes, meat substitutes such as veggie burgers and veggie dogs, tofu (bean curd), eggs (limited to 4–6 per week), nuts (a small handful), and peanut butter (1 tablespoon per day).

Selenium is a mineral that, like vitamins A, E, and C, is an antioxidant, which means that it is vital for long-term protection. Sources of selenium are whole grains, eggs, milk, and garlic. The recommended daily intake of 50–200 mcg is usually found in a vitamin/mineral supplement.

Zinc is a mineral that is lacking in the diets of many older adults. Zinc helps healing and boosts the immune system. The USRDA of 15 mg is found in most vitamin/mineral supplements (be sure the tablet also contains 2 mg of copper, which works with zinc). Since the main food sources of zinc are in protein foods, if you eat adequate protein you are probably getting enough zinc and do not need to supplement your diet unless you are instructed to do so by your doctor.

Proper nutrition keeps us free from disease by bolstering the defenses of the body and by providing the right balance of protein, fat, carbohydrates, and other nutrients. This keeps arteries free from accumulation of fats, maintains normal weight, and protects the vital organs from degeneration. Following are some specific diet-disease relationships and some suggestions for avoiding these problems. These suggestions are not meant to substitute for professional medical advice from your physician. It is vital that you always get qualified medical treatment for any of these problems.

Arthritis

Many factors can contribute to the appearance of arthritis, including heredity, wear and tear on the joints, a malfunctioning immune system, and infections or allergies. In arthritis (and related conditions such as bursitis, tendinitis, and rheumatism), connective tissues in the joints become painfully inflamed. Stiffness and calcification, and eventual deformity, result if the disease is not reversed. Many experts feel that arthritis is related to poor stress competence.

What you can do. Lose excess weight, and then bolster your immune system and meet the increased nutritional requirements of stress with a diet high in B vitamins (particularly pantothenic acid) and vitamin C. Begin each meal with a glass of nutritional yeast (see p. 153). Eat plenty of low-fat or nonfat protein from eggs, dairy products, and dried peas and beans. Extra vitamin E and calcium and magnesium help to prevent stiffening and calcification. One or 2 tablespoons daily of vegetable oils (monosaturates such as olive and canola oil are the best) from salad dressing, or walnuts or almonds, help support hormone production, which is important for keeping painful swelling in check.

Cancer

Cancer is the number two cause of death in the United States (heart disease is number one). People who eat a lot of meat, fat, and sugar, who use tobacco, and who are heavy drinkers have far higher incidences of cancer than those who do not. Deficiencies of vitamins A, C, and E increase cancer risk, as do deficiencies in fiber and the trace mineral selenium.

What you can do. Meat, especially beef, is the primary source of fat in your diet. If you must eat meat, trim off all visible fat, drain off all fat during cooking, and never eat meat gravy or processed meats such as meat hot dogs, lunch meats, and sausage. Do not use meat fat for cooking, and cut back drastically on all fried foods. Replace whole milk and high-fat dairy foods with skim or low-fat milk and cheeses. Eat more fresh fruits and vegetables and whole-grain breads and cereals; they supply fiber, vitamins A, C, and E, and selenium. Stop using tobacco, lose excess weight, and reduce alcohol to under five drinks weekly.

Confusion, Poor Appetite, Depression, and Listlessness

These are symptoms that may or may not be accompanied by aches and pains, but always by irregular breathing patterns. They can often be traced to a poor diet.

What you can do. Consult your doctor first; sometimes these symptoms are signs of an underlying medical problem. If no other problem is found, try improving your diet and practicing your Easy Does It Yoga routine daily. Even two- or three-minute segments, which are so easy to do, will help these problems quickly. Probably the most important thing that you can do, besides eating a well-balanced diet, is to add B-complex vitamins to your diet from nutritional yeast (see p. 153) and other good foods such as whole grains and low-fat or nonfat dairy foods. Remember that the B vitamins are a team, and you must be sure to get some of all of them. If you often don't eat because you are lonely, join a senior center or a support group, or make dates to eat out with friends a few times a week.

Constipation

The primary causes of constipation are a diet low in fiber (roughage), dehydration, and a sedentary lifestyle. Lack of fiber has also been implicated in adding to other problems such as colitis, diverticulosis, and intestinal cancer. Unless they are specifically prescribed by your doctor, avoid using laxatives, as they can be addictive and harmful to your health.

What you can do. Drink 4–6 eight-ounce glasses of nutritious fluids daily. Eat only whole-grain breads and cereals instead of refined-flour products, and try to eat 6–11 servings every day. Eat a variety of fresh fruits and vegetables in at least 3–4 servings per day (for examples of serving sizes, see pp. 149–151). Prune juice, that old remedy, still works. Extra wheat bran in your diet may also be helpful; an easy way to get this is to add it to muffin or bread mixes. Exercise is essential. Every day, do Easy Does It Yoga exercises that compress the abdomen, such as the Knee Squeeze (p. 116). A hint for acid indigestion: Instead of an antacid preparation, try drinking a big glass of buttermilk or nutritional yeast (see p. 153). The protein will neutralize the acids in your stomach and give you a big nutritional boost as well.

Diabetes

Diabetes is a deficiency of the hormone insulin, which is secreted by the pancreas to modulate blood sugar levels. Juvenile diabetes appears in childhood and is not controllable by diet. Our discussion will focus on adult-onset diabetes, which is often brought on by excess weight and a diet too high in sugar, disrupting the body's natural balance of insulin and blood sugar. Diabetics need either to replace insulin by injection or to moderate blood sugar with strict adherence to diet. Most physicians prefer diet management without supplemental insulin, because this treatment causes fewer complications if the patient is compliant with the diet. Some nutritionists believe that a diet high in magnesium, B-complex vitamins, vitamin C, and the trace mineral chromium can reduce insulin needs or restore your own insulin production. Chromium is needed for insulin's effectiveness, and this deficiency may account for many prediabetic conditions.

What you can do. First, you must lose excess weight. Eat small, frequent, well-balanced meals. Important foods to include are eggs, low-fat or nonfat dairy foods, fresh fruits and vegetables, dried peas and beans, and whole-grain breads and cereals. Be sure to make any changes in your diet within the framework of your prescribed diabetic diet. Drink nutritional yeast (see p. 153) before every meal to get high amounts of B vitamins and protein. Nutritional yeast is also a rich source of chromium, a nutrient that helps the body utilize sugar. Three to 5 grams of vitamin C and 400 to 800 IU of vitamin E may also be helpful. Lecithin (in either granular or capsule form) may help to reduce blood fats.

Heart Attacks, Strokes, Hardening of the Arteries, and High Blood Pressure

The typical American diet and lifestyle—a diet too rich in fat and sodium, too little exercise, and poor stress resistance—has made heart disease the number one cause of death. Coronary artery disease, strokes, high blood pressure, hardening of the arteries, memory loss, headaches, dizziness, cold hands and feet, stasis ulcers, gangrene, and poor healing of cuts and broken bones are some of the related conditions associated with a high-fat, high-sodium diet. When my father took high-blood pressure medication, he developed constant diarrhea. After he started taking a high-potency B complex that included folic acid, the diarrhea disappeared and did not return.

What you can do. Get rid of excessive weight. Stop using tobacco completely. Do your Easy Does It Yoga and other exercises every day. Reduce or eliminate meat from your diet, and choose low-fat or nonfat milk, cottage cheese, buttermilk, and nutritional yeast (see p. 153) for extra protein. Limit both butter and margarine, and eat more high-fiber fresh fruits and vegetables. Vitamins A, C, and E help keep your circulatory system healthy, and lecithin (in granular or capsule form) helps the body to reduce blood fats.

Muscle Cramps, Restless Legs, Anxiety, and Insomnia

When the arteries are sluggish due to a high-fat diet, blood can't reach the muscles in the legs and feet to bring them oxygen and calcium. Cramps then result when you exercise the muscles or when your blood pressure naturally drops at night. Most leg cramps, however, are caused by a lack of calcium in the diet.

What you can do. Vitamin E may help increase circulation, and calcium and magnesium can help relax muscle tissue. Increase your consumption of low-fat or nonfat dairy products (especially milk); soy products such as tofu (see p. 152); and dark green, leafy vegetables for extra calcium. Foods rich in vitamin E are wheat germ (sprinkle some on your cereal), unrefined vegetable oils, nuts, and 100 percent whole-grain breads and cereals. New studies suggest that older adults, whose bodies are less efficient at using dietary nutrients, may benefit from supplementing their diet with 200 to 400 IU of vitamin E per day.

Nutritional Anemia

Pallor, depression, and lack of energy and stamina are symptoms of iron deficiency, one of several causes of anemia. Severe folate deficiency anemia (lack of the nutrient folic acid) can cause depression, and is common if there are too few fresh fruits and vegetables in the diet. Deficiencies of vitamins B_6, C, E, or magnesium can also cause anemia.

What you can do. Eat plenty of unrefined foods that are rich in iron, particularly wheat germ; dark green, leafy vegetables; dried fruits; and whole-grain breads and cereals. Good sources of folic acid are fortified cereals, nutritional yeast, lentils and other legumes, and fresh fruits and vegetables.

Obesity

Obesity is becoming an increasing problem in our country. The latest surveys show that, despite the growing abundance of so-called diet foods and low-fat or nonfat products, Americans are steadily gaining weight, not losing it. Over a third of Americans are currently overweight—up from a fourth just twenty years ago. Obesity is usually triggered by increasing inactivity and the naturally changing metabolism of middle age, compounded by a lifetime of poor eating habits. Obesity puts great strain on your heart, lungs, pancreas, and joints, increasing your chances of heart attack, stroke, arthritis, and diabetes.

What you can do. Eat less sugar, fats, and oils, and use low-fat or nonfat dairy products. This means limiting candy, pastry, pies, and cakes, and broiling or baking instead of frying. If you crave sweets, eat fresh or cooked fruits, or try a little sugar-free jam on toast. A severe craving for sweets sometimes indicates a B-vitamin deficiency. Have a nutritional yeast cocktail before every meal. Eat as many fresh fruits and vegetables as you like (served without rich sauces or butter or margarine; try lemon juice and spices instead); dark green, leafy vegetables; and salad vegetables. Limit or cut out alcohol entirely, and replace all soft drinks with seltzer or sparkling water over ice, with lemon or lime (club soda is best avoided because of its sodium content). Avoid the danger of binging by allowing yourself one small sweet thing each day.

Exercise is absolutely essential. If your physician approves, do some form of mild aerobic activity such as walking, swimming, or bicycling at least three times per week. And do your Easy Does It Yoga program every day for the strength, stability, and concentration you need to stay on a healthy weight-loss program.

Osteoporosis

This disease is characterized by weak, brittle bones. It most often affects the hips and back, but can also affect the jawbone and cause teeth to be lost due to gum disease. These problems are caused in part by ingesting too little calcium during one's lifetime. Women lose up to one-third of their bone mass over a lifetime; men about one-fifth.

What you can do. Replace meat with low-fat or nonfat dairy products and eggs. These supply calcium and vitamin D. Drink fluoridated water, and eat whole grains; soy products such as tofu (see p. 152); nuts; and dark green, leafy vegetables, which supply zinc and magnesium. If you already have osteoporosis, ask your doctor or nutritionist about supplementing your diet with extra calcium and magnesium, but don't make that a substitute for getting more calcium and vitamin D from your food. And don't forget to exercise! Studies have shown that regular, moderate exercise of the weight-bearing variety, such as walking or standing Easy Does It Yoga exercises, will help build bone density.

CHAPTER 10

Easy Does It Yoga Philosophy

"My Yoga interest is the first time in my life that I've done something for myself—for me alone."

—Harriet Peel (age 74)

The main result of Yoga is to end separateness, not only within oneself but between oneself and the world. This produces a person who is truly whole, able to face life well fortified with strength and a balanced outlook. This is the powerful product of Yoga philosophy: to stimulate ideas that have meaning in everyday life. It does you no good just to talk about philosophical concepts if you cannot translate them into actions and feelings that help you live a happier, more conscious life. In this chapter, you will find out how Yoga philosophy becomes intricately connected with Yoga practice.

The increased mental control, self-awareness, and concentration that you develop as you practice Yoga will help to alleviate seemingly unshakable feelings of depression, anger, and fear. When you feel emotionally upset, you may have incessant mental conversations, which perpetuate and prolong your distress and sap your energy as well. You can break this destructive cycle by practicing to achieve the detachment that is part of the philosophy of Yoga. You are much more than a body with feelings and a mind. Your body is supported by a great spiritual force that lies deep within you. This spiritual force is like a second body that can merge with your physical body to give you great strength to achieve your goals in life.

Yoga meditation helps to break up cycles of haunting emotional upset by creating a daily habit of a quiet mental vacation that rests the mind. When you return to your everyday concerns, you get a new look at your mind's reaction to them, which gives you a fresh, more effective approach to your problems.

Yoga teaches you how to make your body healthy and beautiful with the least amount of effort. Even if you are severely disabled, Yoga practice will greatly help you to become more comfortable, efficient, and independent. The practical benefits of Yoga practice also include a bright, creative mind, emotional awareness, and sensitivity. You will find relief from boredom, frustration, useless anger, and intolerance. There is no need then to escape into the oblivion of alcohol or drug abuse, or to a fantasy life where you have no contact with the real world.

Yoga is often misinterpreted in the Western world as a religious practice that demands a change of religious observance in the student. Nothing could be further from the truth. Yoga is a strictly individual process that binds the inner emotional being to the outer physical self, producing a whole, strong individual. Yoga has no creed or organized religious observance of any kind. People from any religious background can practice Yoga without fear that their beliefs will be compromised. In fact, most students find that Yoga enhances their life and beliefs by helping them develop a strong, clear, aware, and appreciative outlook on all aspects of their lives.

It is said in the Bhagavad Gita, one of the great books on Yoga, that we are our own best friend and our own worst enemy. As a Yoga student, you learn to become friends with yourself, to stop doing the things that harm your mind and body, and to adjust to the natural changes in body and mind that come to all of us, no matter what our age or physical limitation.

"Now that I'm older and have arthritis in many of my joints, I find that I can't do some of the poses I once did when I was in my twenties—especially in the early morning. At those times, substituting the Easy Does It poses helps me maintain strength, flexibility, and health."

—Jeanetta Ho (age 49)

Yoga philosophy provides a new growth path for anyone who is looking for meaning in life. It is especially effective in later life. It could even be said that the older you get, the better you get; no youngster can come along and leave you in the dust! Supported by the practice of Yogic techniques, the later years can be full of rich discovery, good health, and deep emotional fulfillment.

The practice of Yoga helps us to become stronger, more competent; we can find solutions to our own problems. This new self-reliance can influence our entire community; it is the essence of leadership. People who are healthy, happy, and appreciative of life remain productive and active members of society far longer than do those who feel thwarted by physical limitation. Yoga systems have long been used to supply this growth and expansion.

Age is only one of life's limitations. None of us ever has the perfect body and health that we wish for, yet everyone needs the support of a creative mind and a comfortable outlook. Yoga's remarkable product is showing you how to use whatever body function you have to enhance your mental attitude and thought, no matter what circumstances life has brought your way. Yoga exercises, in fact, were designed to be done in small spaces with the most efficient use of energy and time. This quality makes them ideal for anyone whose mobility is limited. Breathing techniques make sure that circulation is maintained properly, so that the mind remains bright and creative. This is especially important for those enduring enforced inactivity due to a severe illness, recovery, or paralysis.

> *"As a polio survivor, I have to be very selective about the exercise I choose, to avoid muscle exhaustion. Practicing Yoga within my physical limitations has improved my balance and strength and has maintained my flexibility. After a recent bout of pneumonia, the breathing exercises helped me rebuild lung capacity—more oxygen means more energy! Daily meditation staves off the ravages of stress from my professional law practice. My focus and concentration are also enhanced when I practice Yoga; I have improved mental alertness in addition to the physical fitness."*
>
> —Sandra K. Hunter (age 51)

Yoga philosophy, combined with even a few minutes a day of physical practice, produces mental freshness, enabling practitioners to find new strength in themselves. Medication dosages can be reduced, and body functions that seemed to be gone forever often slowly return. One of the greatest benefits is that the practices themselves are so enjoyable that people continue to practice them without the dread of discipline and pain that often accompanies other rehabilitative work.

Probably the greatest realization that comes in Yoga practice is that the body is a vehicle for the expression of an inner spiritual force. When this spiritual force joins with the physical body, it heals the rift of separateness that makes us feel alone and lonely. This creates a whole, balanced person who approaches life with joy and vigor.

Yoga can help you to understand yourself and to find lasting beauty and happiness in yourself, in others, and in the world around you. A great Yogic scholar, Patanjali, taught that in silence, we learn more about the source of ourselves, our thoughts, and our feelings. This is the goal of meditation. As self-control and inner quiet develop, an intensely pleasurable experience of strength and clarity of consciousness begins to grow. When you become really quiet, you are able to experience the real you. There is a lot more in each of us than meets the eye. This is especially important to remember as we get older or when we recover from illness or injury, because many of us devalue ourselves if our bodies do not perform as well as we wish them to.

As we move on in life, it is essential that our minds begin to delve into the more subtle, abstract issues and concepts of both life and death to discover what is lasting and real about ourselves. We are so geared to thinking in terms of products that we have forgotten that wisdom and experience cannot be put in a box and sold. It must be lived, experienced, and transmitted by example. We are not robots all working, as if on an assembly line, to spew out endless items for consumption in the material world. With inner-directed attention, real self-awareness offers new, creative patterns to help us live happier and more productive lives. The materialistic outlook of our society then can be balanced with a mature outlook that recognizes the value and use of intangibles.

"My husband passed away ten years ago. I was depressed for a long time. The Yoga and meditation seem to give me a different viewpoint about life and death. You have to learn to accept things that are in God's hands. My Yoga gives me a tranquil feeling. Somehow, I just feel relaxed and a whole lot happier."

—Jeanne Hrovat (age 66)

FIVE WAYS TO INCREASE PERSONAL GROWTH

Inactivity makes it difficult to keep expanding our mental horizons. The Easy Does It Yoga philosophy, rather than outlining a specific dogma, challenges you to explore perspectives of your own choice. Yoga philosophy awakens a mature acceptance of the limitations of age or disability and inspires an exciting mental challenge that fosters individual growth through the active pursuit of creative thought.

Live in the Present

Try not to dwell in the past. Many of my students have benefited from a simple technique that you can use to help you notice the patterns of thought that repeatedly arise in your mind: Put a small Band-Aid or piece of tape on the inside of your wrist and make a mark on it every time you notice yourself thinking back about how things could have been. Look at your reminder at the end of each day. Being aware of these patterns of thought will help you focus your thoughts on the present.

Learn to live in the present. Decide how you can make today more constructive and satisfying by setting realistic daily goals and step-by-step plans to achieve them. You will encourage self-growth and recognize where you stand, how you feel, and what you want to do today.

Put Ethical Principles into Practice

The ten ethical observances discussed in the classical Yoga literature are considered to be so important that they are listed even before discussions of exercise and meditation! They are: nonviolence, truthfulness, nonstealing, celibacy, nonhoarding, purity, contentment, tolerance, study, and remembrance. Each one of these concepts is a vast reservoir of meaning and interpretation. Our book *Yoga of the Heart* examines each of these ten principles in a separate chapter (see Appendix II).

Nonviolence means not harming yourself or others, not only in the obvious ways, but also more subtly. Do you overindulge in alcohol, caffeine, or sweets? Do you put yourself and others at risk of injury by driving too fast when you are in a hurry?

Truthfulness has to do with keeping your word. Do you always do what you say you are going to do, even in small things? Keeping your word to yourself is a big achievement.

Nonstealing: People feel the need to steal only when they feel lacking in some way. You steal from yourself when you lack concentration; you steal the strength that will help you reach your goals.

Celibacy for periods of time as brief as five minutes a day is an exercise that can be practiced very easily. It gives a new appreciation of the many desires that crowd the mind, and develops a different outlook on love.

Nonhoarding has to do with ownership. In the practice of this ethic, your attitude toward your possessions is much more important than what you own.

Purity is about being 100 percent yourself, unfragmented, strong, and confident. Most of us present different faces to different people; we say one thing and do another; and we are not always clear about who we are or the direction of our life.

Contentment is a state of consciousness. It is the ability to remain in the present moment.

Tolerance is an important characteristic of the hero, who has more than the ordinary ability to withstand life's pressures with steadiness, perseverance, and courage.

Study is an important source of nourishment for the inner self.

Remembrance helps you realize that you are not alone in your quest for self-knowledge. This ethic reminds you of the participation of your unknown inner self.

Exercise your awareness by choosing one of these ethics each week and trying to apply it to your everyday actions and relationships. You can use a wrist tape to note successes and failures. By putting these ideas to the test in your life, you can begin to manifest in your personality the qualities that work for you.

With your friends, form a study group that will give you exciting intellectual challenges. Take adult education courses, take advantage of travel/study programs such as Elderhostel, or just explore some new material at your local library. If you are housebound, find a tutor or ask someone to study with you, and exchange ideas. A knowledge of how other people think and live can be a great support for internal change, especially if you are restricted in physical movement.

Read about various philosophies, religions, mythologies, and psychological concepts, and organize group discussions to share your insights with others. This is especially helpful if you are in recovery from illness, injury, addiction, etc. Some books you might start with include:

Autobiography of a Yogi. Paramahansa Yogananda (Self-Realization Fellowship, 1946). Yogananda was a great Yogi whose teachings had a profound effect on the growth of Yoga in the West. He describes his life and important Yoga concepts in engaging and easy-to-understand terms.

Bhagavad Gita (many translations available). Part of a much longer Indian epic called the Mahabharata, it contains the essence of Yoga philosophy.

The Hero with a Thousand Faces. Joseph Campbell (Princeton University Press, 1949). An investigation of the hero story, which every culture in the world uses to illustrate the individual's search for self-awareness and insight.

The King and the Corpse: Tales of the Soul's Conquest of Evil. Heinrich Zimmer (Princeton University Press, 1957). A wide-ranging examination of several important worldwide myths and their psychological meanings for the individual and the culture as a whole.

Myths to Live By. Joseph Campbell (Bantam Books, 1972). A good general introduction to comparative mythology written by the greatest scholar in this field.

Patanjali and Yoga. Mircea Eliade (Schocken Books, 1969). An in-depth study of classical Yoga as described by the great scholar Patanjali, who lived around A.D. 300.

Philosophies of India. Heinrich Zimmer (Princeton University Press, 1951). In-depth studies of major philosophical influences in India, including Yoga, Brahmanism, Jainism, Buddhism, and others.

Improve Your Mental Health

Mental health results when you harmonize your actions with your thoughts and feelings. Daily meditation will help you clarify your true desires and feelings. With this clarity it will be easy for you to be what you want to be. Practice at least 15 minutes of meditation every day, and always take a few minutes after you are finished to return slowly to your normal thoughts. Notice carefully: How do I feel now?

Seek Out Challenging Relationships

Seek out people and relationships that will give you the opportunity to examine new viewpoints and unfamiliar situations. This will develop flexibility. As you meet these new experiences, try to step back from critical emotional reactions and refrain from making snap judgments that will inhibit communication. Use your wrist tape to record your impulse to judge. If you can open new lines of communication with people who have ideas different from your own, you can comfortably keep pace with rapid societal changes and allow others to benefit from your experience and wisdom.

"I'm thinking differently! I actually am. Is it possible that my thoughts could change? I feel like I'm on a different plane now. I'm not as immature! I was never able to communicate with younger people—I'd start to criticize or find fault or ridicule, and you know, one thing leads to another, and then they'd avoid me because they knew what my reactions always were. I was downright belligerent. Now it seems that if I relax, my mental perception changes and I'm not so critical. I'm smoother and calmer. It surprises me—and them!"

—Helen Gould (age 64)

APPENDIX I

Summary of Research on Easy Does It Yoga

Easy Does It Yoga is a program that consists of specially adapted Yoga exercises—most of which are done in chairs—combined with breathing techniques and relaxation training. All of the techniques are safe and gentle, with endless variations possible according to each individual's physical limitations. *Easy Does It Yoga* includes sections for exercises that can be done in bed, in a wheelchair, or in the pool. A special training program for health professionals or anyone who works with people with physical limitations is presented in our book *The Easy Does It Yoga Trainer's Guide* (see Appendix II).

Researchers in this program in the past twenty years have included:

Durand F. Jacobs, Ph.D., Veterans Administration Medical Center, Loma Linda, California.

Roger N. Hess, Ph.D., Douglas Schultz, Ph.D., and Robert W. Scott, M.D., with the support of a matching grant from the Cleveland Foundation and the American Yoga Association.

David Haber, Ph.D., formerly of the University of South Florida, Tampa, supported by an Administration of Aging Title IV-B research grant and the Older Americans Act, Title III.

Research on the EDY program by the Veterans Administration Medical Center showed strong evidence that simple Yoga techniques can reduce somatic and psychological complaints. Participants being evaluated reported improvements in several areas. Our students found a marked reduction in problems resulting from an unhealthy musculoskeletal system, such as pain in the back, arms, and legs, as well as cramps. In addition, students noticed a general improvement in the functioning of the respiratory system, with less running or bleeding noses, or constant coughing. Many students experienced having an overall improvement of the nervous system. They reported fewer problems of numbness and tingling in the arms and legs, fewer severe headaches, reduced dizziness, and less twitching in the face, head, and shoulder area. Students involved in the program also experienced positive emotional changes. There were marked reductions in anxiety symptoms such as nervousness, irritation, and impulsive behavior. Self-esteem increased, and some older students also reported a renewed interest in sex.

The Cleveland Foundation study explored the effectiveness of the EDY program in augmenting traditional hypertension treatments. Seventy people over the age of fifty-five who suffered mild to moderate hypertension participated in the project. Half of the participants were assigned to the EDY program, and half to a traditional exercise-to-music program. Both groups met twice weekly for 12 weeks. Clinical status was determined before and after the 12 weeks, and was also continued for an additional 12-week follow-up period. Both the EDY program and exercise-to-music program led to reductions in blood pressure, with the Yoga program participants experiencing a statistically significant change. Both groups lost some weight, though neither was significant. Both groups reduced pulse rate significantly over the entire 24-week period. A 29-item symptoms checklist included anxiety, depression, tiredness, nervousness, trouble sleeping, stiff joints, and muscle weakness. Results of the symptoms checklist for every comparison in the two groups showed improvement among the Yoga students, which was sustained over the follow-up period. For the exercise-to-music group, although there was some improvement in all areas, only two of the differences were significant, and both of them appeared only at the end of the follow-up period. In summary, both programs led to an improvement in physical well-being, but the Yoga training resulted in a greater feeling of general well-being.

Two senior centers in west-central Florida were chosen for an exploratory study, supported by the Administration of Aging, to evaluate the use of Yoga as a preventive health care program. The study was community based, using white volunteers at the SS Center, and black volunteers at the JJ Center. At each site older persons were equally distributed between a Yoga class and another activity, such as a film series or an art class. Classes were held once a week for 10 weeks at a community site, with daily homework assignments by the students on their own at home. Compared to other group programs with minority elders, dropout rates were quite low. Yoga participants reduced their systolic blood pressure level in comparison to control persons at the SS Center at the .09 level of significance. Yoga participants at the JJ Center did not lower blood pressure levels in comparison to control persons. Among SS Yoga participants, self-assessed health status improved, as did psychological well-being, in comparison to the other group. At the JJ Center, Yoga participants did not improve on the self-assessed health status measurement or the psychological well-being scale in comparison to the other group. Though equivalent procedures were implemented at both centers, black older students were not motivated to practice Yoga on their own at home. While older students at both centers attended the weekly class on a regular basis, the SS participants practiced Yoga an additional five times per week on average, while the JJ participants practiced only one additional time per week on average. It was concluded that the psychological response to Yoga in the black community might need to improve before the potential benefits of Yoga with regard to high blood pressure or hypertension could be determined. One future direction for low-income minority elders is to increase class contact from one to three or four times a week. Some analysts believe that more frequent direct leadership with minority elders is necessary to encourage them to intervene on their own behalf.

The Older Americans Act (Title III) provided funding for a recreation-fitness program for older rural and urban residents of Florida's Tampa Bay area. Just over 100 people, divided into two groups, participated in independent, controlled studies of the impact of Easy Does It Yoga on physical and emotional health. Group I consisted of predominantly white, middle-class female high school graduates living with their spouses, and Group II was nearly one-half black, predominantly female, middle- to lower-class, junior high school graduates. Within each group about half the participants were randomly assigned to the EDY treatment group, and the other half to the control group. A battery of tests was given to assess the frequency of somatic and nonsomatic complaints (Hopkins Symptom Checklist), to ascertain present levels of tension and nervousness (Spielberger's State Trait Anxiety Inventory), to ascertain present feelings of self-worth (Rosenberg's Self-Esteem Scale), to measure opinions about feelings of accomplishment (Neugarten's Life Satisfaction Index), and to monitor blood pressure. Additional demographic and health care behavior variables were measured. Also, measurements were recorded for the average number of minutes per day and days per week that the Yoga techniques were performed at home. The results of Group I test battery scores showed that the EDY group outperformed the control group on every measure except the somatic and nonsomatic complaints. In addition, all changes in mean scores for the EDY group were positive, except for the life satisfaction score. However, the indicated decrease in life satisfaction was 50 percent greater for the control group. Test scores for Group II showed that the EDY group did better on every measure compared to the control group. Group I participants practicing the EDY regimen of exercise, breathing, relaxation, and meditation techniques at home reported practicing an average of 35 minutes per day. In Group II, EDY participants practiced an average of 32 minutes per day.

APPENDIX II

Resources from the

American Yoga Association

For further information on Yoga, including a complete catalog of the books and tapes described below, please send a self-addressed envelope stamped with postage for two ounces to:

American Yoga Association
P.O. Box 19986
Sarasota, Florida 34276
Telephone: (941) 927-4977
Fax: (941) 921-9844
E-mail: Yogamerica@aol.com
Website: http://users.aol.com/amyogaassn

We offer classes in the Cleveland, Ohio, area. For more information, write or call:

American Yoga Association
P.O. Box 18105
Cleveland Heights, Ohio 44118
Telephone: (216) 556-1313

BOOKS

The American Yoga Association Beginner's Manual (Fireside/Simon & Schuster, 1987). Complete instructions for more than ninety Yoga exercises and breathing techniques; also includes three ten-week curriculum outlines and chapters on nutrition, philosophy, stress management, sports, and pregnancy.

The American Yoga Association's New Yoga Challenge (Contemporary Books, 1997). The chapters in this book—on Attention, Energy, Strength, Flexibility, Steadiness, and Focus—introduce different approaches for achieving oneness of body and mind through challenging physical workouts and creative philosophical concepts. The concluding chapter, "The Powerful Individual," shows you how to design your own routine to suit your needs, goals, and tendencies.

The American Yoga Association Wellness Book (Kensington Books, 1996). A basic routine to maintain health and well-being, plus chapters on how Yoga can specifically help fifteen common health conditions, among them arthritis, heart disease, back pain, PMS, menopause, weight management, insomnia, and headaches.

Conversations with Swami Lakshmanjoo, Volume I: Aspects of Kashmir Shaivism (American Yoga Association, 1995). Edited transcripts of Alice Christensen's interviews with Swami Lakshmanjoo, talking about his childhood and early years in Yoga, plus some basic concepts in the philosophy of Kashmir Shaivism.

Conversations with Swami Lakshmanjoo, Volume II: The Yamas and Niyamas of Patanjali (American Yoga Association, 1998). Edited transcripts of Alice Christensen's dialogs with Swami Lakshmanjoo about these essential ethical guidelines in Yoga.

The Easy Does It Yoga Trainer's Guide (Kendall/Hunt, 1995). A complete beginner's manual for teaching the Easy Does It Yoga program to seniors or others with physical limitations. Excellent for health professionals, activities directors, physical therapists, home health aides, and others who work with the elderly or in rehabilitative services.

The Joy of Celibacy (Forthcoming). This book examines how the unconscious is influenced by the sexual sell of modern advertising and suggests a five-minute celibacy break to help build awareness and self-knowledge.

The Light of Yoga (American Yoga Association, 1997, rev. ed.). A chronicle of the unusual circumstances that catapulted Alice Christensen into Yoga practice in the early 1950s, including the teachers and experiences that shaped her first years of study.

Meditation (American Yoga Association, 1994). A collection of excerpts from Alice Christensen's lectures and classes on the subject of meditation, including a section of questions and answers from students.

Reflections of Love (American Yoga Association, 1995). A collection of excerpts from Alice Christensen's lectures and classes on the subject of love.

20-Minute Yoga Workouts: The Perfect Program for the Busy Person (Ballantine, 1995). Brief routines that anyone can fit into the busiest schedule. Includes chapters on women's issues, toning and shaping, the "20-minute challenge," and workouts to do when you're away from home.

Yoga of the Heart: Ten Ethical Principles for Gaining Limitless Growth, Confidence, and Achievement (Daybreak/Rodale Books, 1998). An in-depth discussion of how practicing the subtle aspects of Yoga's essential ethics—nonviolence, truthfulness, nonstealing, periods of celibacy, nonhoarding, purity, contentment, tolerance, study, and remembrance—can help an individual welcome the spiritual body that resides within.

AUDIOTAPES

Complete Relaxation and Meditation with Alice Christensen (American Yoga Association, 1992). A two-tape audiocassette program that features three guided meditation sessions of varying lengths, including instruction for a seated posture, as well as a discussion of meditation experiences.

The "I Love You" Meditation Technique (American Yoga Association, 1995). This technique begins with the experience of a more conscious connection with the breath through love. It then extends this feeling throughout the body and mind in relaxation and meditation. This tape teaches you the beauty of loving yourself and removes unseen fear.

VIDEOTAPES

Basic Yoga (Peter Pan Industries/Parade Video, 1993). A complete introduction to Yoga that includes exercise, breathing, and relaxation and meditation techniques. Provides detailed instruction in all the techniques including variations for more or less flexibility, plus a special limbering routine and back-strengthening exercises. Features a 30-minute practice session in a Yoga class setting for a convenient routine to do daily.

Conversations with Swami Lakshmanjoo (American Yoga Association). A set of three videotapes in which Alice Christensen introduces Swami Lakshmanjoo and talks with him about his background, the philosophy of Kashmir Shaivism, and other topics in Yoga. (Some material corresponds to volume I of the book *Conversations with Swami Lakshmanjoo*.)

The Hero in Yoga: A Videotape Study Program (American Yoga Association). A series of twenty-four videotaped lectures by Alice

Christensen on Joseph Campbell's landmark text *The Hero with a Thousand Faces,* showing how the adventure of the hero, represented in mythologies all over the globe, parallels the Yoga student's search for self-actualization.

The Yamas and Niyamas: A Videotape Study Program (American Yoga Association). A series of twenty-five videotapes of Alice Christensen's comprehensive lectures on the ethical guidelines that form the cornerstone of Yoga philosophy and practice.

Nutrition Resources

Eat Right, Live Longer. Neal Barnard, M.D. (Harmony Books, 1995). An eight-step program for using a healthy diet to counteract the aging process.

Get Healthy Now! With Gary Null: A Complete Guide to Prevention, Treatment, and Healthy Living. Gary Null (contributor), Amy McDonald (editor) (Seven Stories Press, 1999).

Jane Brody's Nutrition Book: A Lifetime Guide to Good Eating for Better Health and Weight Control by the Personal Health Columnist of the New York Times. Jane E. Brody (Bantam Doubleday Dell, 1989).

Let's Stay Healthy: A Guide to Lifelong Nutrition (New American Library/Dutton, 1983) and *Let's Get Well* (Harcourt, Brace & World, 1965). Adelle Davis's books are so well researched and written that nutritionists still use her books as a reference even though decades have passed since her first book came out in the mid-1960s. She includes much general information about all essential nutrients as well as common health problems, and describes how nutritional changes can help.

Nutrition Action. Monthly newsletter published by the Center for Science in the Public Interest, Suite 300, 1875 Connecticut Avenue NW, Washington, DC 20009-5728. Contains up-to-date information about research in nutrition as well as feature articles about current issues or commonly asked questions.

Walnut Acres (mail-order firm for nutritional yeast and other natural foods). Penns Creek, PA 17862; (800) 433-3998.

INDEX

ABOUT THE AMERICAN YOGA ASSOCIATION

The American Yoga Association teaches a comprehensive and balanced program of Yoga exercise, breathing, and meditation. Rather than focusing primarily on physical conditioning, our core curriculum acknowledges the deeper possibilities of Yoga and encourages the inner-directed awareness that eventually leads to greater self-knowledge. This reliance on individual experience and feeling is a central theme in the science of Yoga, and it underlies the philosophical system of Kashmir Shaivism, which supports our line of teaching.

ABOUT THE AUTHOR

Alice Christensen is a Yoga teacher with the rare ability to make the often complex ideas and techniques of Yoga accessible to our Western outlook and lifestyle. In 1968, she established the American Yoga Association, then the first and only nonprofit organization in the United States dedicated to education in Yoga.

Alice has consistently presented Yoga in a clear, classical manner for over forty years. She presents Yoga without dogma or prescription, as a potent avenue for individual inquiry, in formats that can be used to enhance any lifestyle. Whether the goal is to maintain health or to explore the nature of the self, her programs can be used to achieve a wide range of goals.